Forew

Dr Andrew
St George's Hospital Medical Sch.   ..versity of London

This book is the result of a mother's search for answers to the distressing symptoms suffered by her child, and so many readers may expect a partisan and unscientific work. What emerges, however, is far from this. The author has listened carefully to many mothers and taken seriously what they say (something some of us supposedly learnt as medical students). Despite no formal medical or scientific training, she has read more widely than many experts and tested parents' observations against the scientific literature. She has then sought out specialists with differing backgrounds and views and posed many pertinent questions as well as taking note of their opinions and occasional words of caution. The result is a sound and sympathetic approach to food intolerance and infant feeding which is easy to read and tackles both theory and practice. Her frank and at times provocative questioning of established dogma will refresh some and trouble others; but orthodox doctors, practitioners of alternative medicine and politicians all receive a fair share of often justifiable criticism. Some of the conclusions drawn may not withstand the test of time, but others may prove to be more significant than is presently realized; this is inevitable when dealing with a controversial and confusing topic such as food allergy. In no way does this detract from this extremely useful book which will be a help to parents and should live up to its title as far as the 'experts' are concerned.

Foreword

Professor J. W. Gerrard,
Department of Paediatric Allergy, University of Saskatchewan

As a result of her own experience and that of other nursing mothers whom she has helped, coupled with her wide reading, Maureen Minchin has acquired an excellent understanding of diet-related problems encountered in infants and young children. Some of her comments are speculative, but this is understandable, for our knowledge in this field is still incomplete, but her fundamental advice is sound, and the sooner it is implemented the better for the next generation of babies. Nursing mothers, particularly if they come from an allergic background, and many family physicians, paediatricians, and obstetricians will all have much to learn from *Food for Thought*.

Foreword

G. J. Ebrahim,
Reader of Tropical Child Health, Institute of Child Health, London

During my ten years as the only paediatrician in Tanzania I discovered that mother's milk is the newborn's best insurance for survival. Diarrhoea in the breast-fed infant was rare, and other infective illnesses, if they occurred, were less serious. In those who developed diarrhoea at the time of weaning, hypernatraemia was rare. In fact during my entire stay in Tanzania I scarcely, if ever, made a diagnosis of hypernatraemia (too much sodium in the blood) in a child with diarrhoea, whereas the medical journals were at the time full of accounts of the condition indicating its prevalence and seriousness as experienced in some of the major West European centres. Was I missing a serious condition?

Today the medical journals no longer discuss hypernatraemia and its incidence has declined markedly. Before that medical texts used to give vivid description of hypercalcaemia (too much calcium in the blood). This condition has also virtually disappeared, which means that both hypernatraemia and hypercalcaemia in infants are preventable, or should one be more honest and describe them as iatrogenic, that is, caused by the treatment—in this case bottle-feeding. However, much we may rejoice in the disappearance of these two conditions that fact does remain that a proportion of children either died or were permanently damaged on account of them. We now know that both the conditions were caused by a faulty diet offered to an individual at an age when the body's physiological defences are least able to cope with it. Infancy and childhood is such a vulnerable period and the denial of a natural food viz. mother's milk carries the potential risk of disease. The risk arises not only from the loss of the protection which breast milk provides but also because of the extraneous substances that may be present in the formulae offered. Most of us do not appreciate that a large proportion of the so-called modern formulae are further removed from milk, of any variety, than we think. What are the dangers of exposing the newborn's gut to

Foreword

cotton-seed oil, coconut oil, maize oil, or soya fat? How do these substances affect gut responses especially the release of gut hormones? Are our extraction processes so reliable that not even a trace of other constituents of those substances or carrier molecules of extracting agents do not contaminate the oil obtained?

Food additives and colouring matter have become a part of daily eating in most industrial societies. The average adult in the industrial world consumes daily a quantity of preservatives equal in amount to five tablets of aspirin! No-one would want to do so knowingly, leave aside expose the young ones to such risks. The fact is that the food industry must be more open and provide details to the consumers. If such details about contents and processing are not voluntarily forthcoming then consumer organizations will have to wring them out of the industry. This is especially necessary with regard to the present diversity of 'junk' foods.

This book is about thoughtful eating. It is possible for all of us to feed ourselves and our families on healthy foods which are not all that difficult to prepare, and in the long run much cheaper. The author has assembled a considerable amount of useful information on food, and especially on the dangers of convenience foods. The book is full of good common sense and a great deal of effort has gone into making it available at a low cost. I have no doubt that this new edition will enjoy the same popularity as it predecessors.

Contents

Contents

Introduction

This book is the result of a process of dialogue. It has grown out of parental experience, nurtured by interested medical professionals and others. It has been tested—in so far as any such theories can be tested—against the experience of what must now be thousands of people. However, it is important that you, the reader, understand both the origins and basis of the book, so that you can appreciate its strengths and weaknesses. I would ask only of you, 'not the will to believe, but the wish to find out', which, as someone said, is the exact opposite.

In 1976 I interrupted an Oxford postgraduate scholarship to have children—and experienced at first hand the nightmare of infantile colic and the many problems of mismanaged breast-feeding. My research interests switched abruptly from medical history to infant nutrition and development. The literature proved more helpful than the myriad advisers—professional and lay—that I had consulted.

Within a few months my local infant welfare sister was asking me to visit mothers with problem babies, as she recognized that I had solved many problems which she was unable to help with. Those women, and others in parent groups I became involved with, were crucial to the birth of this book. Like myself, many were confident professionals who had chosen to have children, and were not easily put off by glib explanations that crying babies were 'normal', or that professional women made over-anxious mothers who somehow produced colicky infants. (Of course, if the women were young and insecure, it was their inexperience that caused the baby's problems—as one woman wisely said at one meeting, 'you can't win—you're either too young or too old'.) As a woman who saw those women in their own homes with their babies, I could not write them off as tense, unreliable observers. They weren't.

It was a radiologist who first noted the link between her intake of cows' milk and colic in her breast-fed son. This was confirmed many times in other cases. It was clear that cows' milk was not the sole or even chief dietary problem for some—foods incriminated ranged from nuts and yeast supplements to sugary 'junk foods', tea, and coffee.

Food for thought

In trying to establish why some children were affected and others not, the only connection immediately apparent was that all severely colicky babies had been given bottles of artificial formulae in hospital—a practice that many mothers protested against even then. Primiparous mothers were and are especially likely to have their babies 'comp'-ed—given complementary feeds of milk formulae—but not all the children were first born. In some cases mothers had had other 'placid' children at another hospital, and then had a 'colicky' one at a hospital where 'comps' were routine. These mothers were especially vehement in their rejection of the prevalent idea that colic is somehow created by mother–child interaction and tension.

The colic–food-intolerance question was and is just one aspect of my concern about infant nutrition. In fact, I have spent and spend more time studying general breast-feeding issues of many kinds. However, as my son Philip outgrew colic my memory of that nightmare did not fade. I tried to make sure that my next child was not given complementary formula, and was rewarded with an angelic baby who was sheer delight to live with, and a great boost for my self-image as a mother. (Crying babies are so demoralizing, until you realize that it really is some external problem, and not your fault.) In addition, I read all I could, and listened to mothers, and asked question of professionals.

By late 1979 I felt sufficiently confident to raise the issue publicly. The result was an article on colic published in the August 1980 *NMAA Newsletter*. The response surprised everyone involved. Women wrote from all over Australia, either to:

— express their thanks, as their 'comp'-ed baby was no longer screaming after elimination of cows' milk from maternal and/or infant diet;
— insist that 'comp' feeds could *not* be responsible, as their exclusively breast-fed babies were colicky too. (Investigation of these cases usually suggested that the babies had been sensitized *in utero* by maternal binges, or due to abnormal intestinal permeability in food- and inhalant-intolerant mothers.)

All of these mothers were followed up. Almost all are still corresponding; almost all now have children medically diagnosed

Introduction

as food-intolerant. Some examples may be found in the case histories.

The result of that first article was a follow-up article in January 1981, and 800 copies of a 40-page summary of what parents and the research seemed to be saying. This also became the basis of a detailed submission, in December 1981, to the National Health and Medical Research Council, which resulted in the formation of a working party on food intolerance, whose report was published in October 1984.

Response from parents continued to grow, so that the 40-page summary grew into a book. Being by then certain that I had hit upon a major, unrecognized social problem, I saw no need to seek commercial publication. Instead I published it in July 1982 with the help of my husband and friends—and 5000 copies disappeared in a few months; another 6000 sold in the next six months—without any commercial distribution. That fact, and other aspects of public response, made it quite clear that thousands of normal, 'healthy' Australian families had been suffering from the effects of food, chemical, and inhalant intolerances for many years. Here in Australia the book is still selling well—another 11 000 of a revised and expanded edition have been sold since July 1983.

It seemed to me highly likely that all Western countries would have similar problems on a similar scale, owing to the abandonment of breast-feeding and the increasing chemical burden environmentally, as well as other factors. It also seemed to me that all international health bodies ought to be aware of the extraordinary findings reported by otherwise healthy, sensible, privileged Australian families, since socioeconomic deprivation could only compound some of these problems. Hence from the very beginning I sent hundreds of copies around the world to groups and individuals concerned with maternal and child health, as well as academic and clinical researchers. Response from the experts was most encouraging. Several English researchers urged me to consider publication in the United Kingdom—so on a study tour in October 1983 I contacted Oxford University Press—and hence this edition. Royalties from UK sales will go to Child Health Matters, a group supplying books to health workers in countries where exchange problems make it difficult to buy books. This arises from my concern to remain credible in a world filled with

Food for thought

people making a great deal of money out of health and sickness—whatever defects the book may have, it is written out of conviction rather than any desire to cash in on the 'newest fad'.

I hope that history will made a few things clear. Firstly, that this has been and is a collaborative process. Your input could be of value to other parents. If you read this, find it works or find it doesn't, consider this section inadequate or that one overdone—say so. I guarantee that your ideas will be taken seriously, weighed against other parents' responses and the literature, and the next edition will be shaped in some way by your experience too. I cannot stress too highly that the primary basis of this book is the ordinary experience of Australian parents. None of us invented our problems after reading the literature—rather, we compared notes and to our amazement recognized that our problems were similar. Finding a respectable literature supporting our observations was an unexpected bonus—unexpected because in 1976 few of our doctors or nurses seemed to be aware that such medical evidence existed. Your observations of your family can be of tremendous use: no one knows them, or you, as well.

Secondly, you should understand that this subject has been and is controversial and that this book is not without its critics. As I have said in all previous versions, 'This book is designed as a summary of what seem to be reliable medical writings, and is based on the experience of scores of parents. However, the whole field of food-intolerance is so much under-researched that some of what is written is bound to be disproved at a later date. I do not, therefore, urge parents to accept what is written as authoritative, much less infallible. I would like it to be seen as a very preliminary attempt at providing practical preventive and therapeutic advice. The ideas proposed have been very helpful to some parents—helpful in identifying the true nature of the family's problems; in modifying, eliminating, or preventing symptoms; and in encouraging parents to seek skilled specialist help'.

None of the criticism to date has been unexpected, and almost all of it has been both constructive and fair-minded. (Only a tiny fraction was intemperate and dogmatic.) Wherever possible I have worked the comments into the text of this edition, strengthened existing warnings and added new ones. So make sure you read the book carefully and heed those warnings. Never act until you have thought through what you plan to do, and have taken all possible

Introduction

precautions. If in doubt, seek further information before you act. This is a serious business. Every year there are cases of children and adults dying of what are mostly preventable allergic reactions.

It is undoubtedly that, and the fact that some malnourished people have been on prolonged elimination diets, which prompted a very few professionals to suggest that such information ought not be made available to parents without constant medical supervision, for fear it may be misused. Of course it can be, and despite all my warnings, probably will be by some—just as many misuse and misinterpret their doctor's prescriptions, chemical and verbal. If you, as a parent, think such information is valuable, take care not to lend weight to such criticism. Try to communicate your difficulties to your GP, who will probably be quite interested once he realizes the substantial basis of these ideas. Indeed, many of my best customers are GPs, chemists, and even consultant allergists and other specialists, who order dozens of copies because it saves 'me from repeating myself *ad nauseam* for the next few years', as one put it!

Thirdly, its history means that this book is very much geared towards fairly literate readers. It is not the best book available for some parents—but I hope that its bibliography will point out which books are best suited to particular groups. I don't have the time or the skills to write as other than an educated professional. My concern is to convince professionals and other community opinion leaders, that is the people who have power to change things, for themselves and for the powerless. However, in saying that, I am not engaging in the commonplace habit of denigrating the intelligence of 'ordinary' parents. It is my experience that given sufficient motivation and the most basic literacy skills, parents are capable of following extremely complex subjects. So I try to write clearly and directly without over-simplifying too much. To make an informed decision has to mean being aware of complexity, alas.

Fourthly, because of the help I have received from the medical profession, I am not trying to encourage do-it-yourself medicine. I am trying to encourage do-it-together medicine. Although many parents have unfortunately found that skilled medical help is not as widely available as it ought to be, I would continue to urge them, within limits of distance and income, to find receptive doctors, whether GP, allergist, gastroenterologist, paediatrician, or whoever. Contact a parent self-help allergy group for suggestions if you are desperate. But remember that doctors are human, and constantly learning—and they need your feedback (see p. 77).

It must be acknowledged that there are problems inherent in publicizing these ideas at this point in time. In the absence of numerous rigorous studies of the effect of restricting or eliminating dietary antigens in pregnancy and lactation and for the neonate, it cannot be said that the suggestions made are proven to be widely valid—in the fairly narrow 'scientific' meaning of proof. I therefore run the risk of alarming some, or making life difficult for the family cooks— and perhaps making 'proof' difficult for lack of willing subjects! Such concerns must be balanced against the possibility of continued widespread lifelong harm to infants and families—either directly, or as a consequence of the child's difficulties. (If a baby cries for months, and is constantly dirty, the best of mothers will come close to breakdown or battering, to mention but two common outcomes.) I have become convinced that the latter risks are far graver, and the need imperative, even for inadequate help.

In reaching that conclusion there was one decisive factor. It is this: none of the suggestions for change is positively harmful in itself. Even my most intemperate critics have failed to make any specific criticisms of what I have said: they usually insist that what I have said will be misinterpreted or misused by stupid or careless readers. Many suggestions are simply a matter of common sense. Some have proven positive benefits. I would hope that the general result would be:

(1) to make parents more conscious of the need for good balanced nutritional habits in themselves and their children, and to suggest further reading;

(2) to encourage doctors and nurses to take parents more seriously when they report curious observations about their child's diet, health, and behaviour; and to refer parents to skilled specialists if they themselves cannot help;

(3) to persuade hospitals to review procedures and practices which have not been, and possibly never can be, shown to be beneficial to parents or children—and to relearn the largely forgotten art of the successful management of lactation.

During the process of revisions, I have been under various pres-

Introduction

sures to be more/less favourable to the present party lines of orthodox/alternative medicine; more/less critical of doctors/patients—and so on. My emphases change as I am presented with evidence which changes my thinking. But my basic position is that of a parent making sense of this problem primarily from the experience of my own and many other families. That necessarily means being independent of all current parties, as parents find benefits in, and problems with, virtually all the current therapies. I believe this to be a useful and very practical perspective for all practitioners to be aware of—especially those who practise not as community physicians but as specialists in research establishments. One hears from some of these such dogmatic statements of faith about what the incidence of these problems 'should be' in the community—statements which lack historical or cultural perspective and yet are believed, and taken as proof of 'over-diagnosis' requiring stricter management by (of course) specialists, not GPs. Other such experts publicly describe a diagnosis of hyperactivity as 'mischievous', then go on to make further statements of belief about the 'real' problem being parental expectations, maternal interaction, or whatever. (A more damaging and unscientific diagnosis would be hard to imagine.)

Such people need constant exposure to parental reality. Since their own patients are often much too overawed to question, talk back, or protest at either diagnosis or prescribed therapy, I would ask them to read this book. They may not agree with some of it, but they should know more about what patients *are* thinking and feeling. And if they do not agree, I would welcome contrary evidence or a chance or discuss our points of disagreement. I am certain that there is much (in both content and style) to annoy such specialists, who are used to the careful language of science, with its determined neutrality. None the less, as professionals they should be able to stand apart from their irritations and learn from parental experience—and, I hope, allow us to learn from theirs.

As before, responsibility for the contents of this book remains mine alone. Although I have worked closely with many different groups, this book is written by me in my private capacity. The ideas expressed therein are my own as far as that is possible in today's world. The mention of any groups or individuals may signify that I approve of them. It does not necessarily signify that they approve of the ideas in this book. Further, while I have done my best to ensure that the information in this book is accurate and the recommended procedures are safe, I cannot be held responsible for the consequences of their use or misuse by those who fail to consult qualified medical advisers. You are individual; your health is your responsibility. I hope this book helps you make more informed decisions about your family's health.

How this book is organized

The first part of this book is a general overview of the problem of food intolerance, organized under subheadings, usually in the form of questions commonly asked. The second part is a compilation of practical advice from various sources. Please do not go to that second part and use it out of context, without reading this earlier discussion. While the suggestions therein are the best that have been made available to me, very few researchers are publishing much about prevention and practical help. You need to understand the whole, including problems, before taking up any one part. And the last part is self-explanatory.

Some people involved in the genesis of this book

Dr Mavis Gunther, whose book *Infant feeding* saved my sanity, solved my breast-feeding problems, and quite possibly preserved my children from serious disease. Without her work through the breast-feeding 'Dark Ages' none of my researches would have begun. My own mother, who breast-fed all her children and took it for granted that I would breast-feed mine, despite any difficulties. My own health, and my children's, probably owes a great deal to her action and commonsense. My husband Jim, for his constant assistance and encouragement, and our three children, who have taught me just how charming, independent, and lively normal healthy children are. All those Australian families, friends, relations, and professionals, acknowledged in previous editions. Andy Beckingham, who has helped me adapt this very Australian book for an English audience. Richard Seel and Alison Spiro of the National Childbirth Trust (NCT)'s Breast-feeding Promotion Group for their contributions. Professor Maurice Lessof, Dr G. Ebrahim, Dr Andrew Cant, and many others who have advised, criticised, encouraged, and supported me despite my lack of medical qualifications.

To all these people, my affectionate thanks.

Introduction

My thanks also to the following for permission to use copyright material, noted in the text: AIA, Canada; AHRTAG, London; Dr W. Crook, Dr G. J. Ebrahim, London; Professor R. Hamburger, California; Dr R. Mackarness, now of Melbourne; Macmillan Press Ltd., Methuen & Co. Pty. Ltd.; *Modern Medicine* (UK); Plenum Press, New York; Professor D. Rapp, New York; The Royal College of Physicians of London; Dr D. Stigler, Denver; Sun Books, Melbourne; Alan Foley, Pty. Ltd., Sydney; *The Lancet*, London.

The pressing need to prevent the spread of unnecessarily artifical feeding in developing countries should not deflect us from awareness of our profound ignorance of the effect such changes may have had in developed countries. Immunological theory can suggest that many adverse effects, early and late, may arise from deprivation or inactivation of maternal protective systems, perhaps especially in some vulnerable individuals. *The only rational deduction is that such a physiological system should be left undisturbed, unless unavoidable, until we know for certain that it is safe to do so.*

Professor J.S. Soothill, in *Immunology of infant feeding* (ed. A.W. Wilkinson), Plenum Press, New York (1981).

PART 1

Discussion of food intolerance

1

Food intolerance

If a friend says, 'I'm allergic to eggs', we all have a rough idea of what he means. When he eats eggs, or in some cases even touches or smells them, his body reacts in a strange and (usually) unpleasant way. 'Allergy', to most people, means any adverse or altered bodily reaction to a foreign substance touched, smelt, inhaled, eaten, or injected. This in fact is the original meaning of the word, as carefully defined by its inventor, von Pirquet, who wanted a word which made no judgment about *how* that strange reaction came about.[1]

Some professionals nowadays are more discriminating. 'Allergy' has been more strictly defined to mean only those altered bodily reactions currently known to involve the body's immune system. Classifications of allergy exist,[2] labelling the type of allergic response, according to the time and type of bodily effect, etc. What the general public calls allergy, some professionals would label intolerance, or hypersensitivity, or idiosyncrasy—until it has been definitely linked with an 'abnormal' immune response, or an exaggerated one. This change of terminology is relatively recent, and not yet completely standardized, but it explains why many doctors insist that coeliac disease, for example, is not an allergy, when the patient, who knows that certain foods cause symptoms, still thinks that it is. 'Intolerance' is the broader, less precise term, meaning abnormal reactivity by the body. 'Allergy' is one variety of bodily intolerance—the one that involves the immune system. And there are many different immune responses.

WHAT HAPPENS IN AN IMMUNE REACTION (OR 'ALLERGY')?

This next piece is the only really complicated bit in the book. You do not have to understand immune reactions in great detail in

---

[1] Raised numbers refer to Notes at the end of the book (pp. 234–42).

Food for thought

order to deal with the problems they pose. However, it does help many parents to feel that they have some idea of the nature of the reactions involved. That being so, a little detail is here. Don't worry if this seems off-putting—you can come back to this section later if need be. The diagram on p. 6 is a very much simplified outline of some of the things that happen in an allergic response. For you need to understand that different things happen, depending on the type of response and the parts of the immune system that are involved. The body recognizes and rejects any foreign (non-self) substances that find their way to where they shouldn't be, from the transplant to the virus. Problems with food and inhalant particles or breakdown products are just another aspect of the workings of our immune system, which we all depend upon to protect us from infection or other foreign invasion. But in any complex system, minor defects can arise due either to inherited factors or environmental ones, or both. The food-intolerant person, for instance, may be born with low levels of immunoglobulin A (IgA) which protects his gut; he may be bottle-fed and so fail to receive IgA in his mother's milk; and, because bottle-fed (with pathogenic bacteria therefore colonizing his gut), he may develop gastroenteritis which causes injury to his gut lining. It may take one of these factors, or all three, to bring about an allergy to cow's milk. The original immune deficiency is an important defect, but it might not have led to allergic reactions by itself. And of course everybody is different in this as in other ways, across a wide range that is considered 'normal'.

Much basic work remains to be done concerning the body's immune system, even though immunology has expanded enormously in the last decade. A rough outline of what is thought to happen in some immune reactions is as follows.[3]

Stage one: primary inflammatory response

Some substance gets into the body by any one of a number of routes—skin, nose and throat, mouth. There it is recognized as non-self, or foreign; it excites a response. The primary response is to attempt to engulf the foreign material. The inflammation that occurs simultaneously allows more white cells to pass from the blood-vessels to the site of the 'invasion' and it is these white cells which attempt to engulf the foreigner. If they eliminate the intruder, the inflammation subsides and all is well. The same pro-

4

Food intolerance

cess occurs with a cut finger, a sore throat, or a bout of mastitis—foreignness excites inflammation.

Stage two: specific immune response

Sometimes, however, the invader is not eliminated but altered by this process. Here the specific immune response begins. It involves:

(1) the formation of antibodies or immunoglobulins (IgE, IgM, IgG, IgA, IgD) which are tailor-made to fit a specific invader, or excitant. (This excitant may or may not be classed as an antigen.[4])

(2) the creation of cell-mediated, delayed hypersensitivity and elimination of excitants or antigens.

Normally the antibodies and cells between them destroy and eliminate the antigen—and so people recover from viral or bacterial invasion. The antibodies, once created to combat that specific antigen, remain within the body, and the creation of more is faster on a second challenge. This is the principle on which mass vaccination programmes are based—once a child has been vaccinated against a mild form of a disease, he can cope better with the real disease because he already has antibodies to it. This is *immunity*.

Stage three: allergy

If the antigen is not yet eliminated, further reactions are evoked. These are the allergic reactions, types I–IV. The persistence of the antigen may be due to inherited deficiencies in the immune system, or to the continued ingestion of the antigen, or some other unknown factor. The allergic response is harmful to the body, and produces symptoms that may or may not be recognizable as a specific disease. To some degree this depends on which part of the body manifests symptoms—the 'target organ'.

In some people, specific antibodies are located on mast cells in the body's mucous surfaces or connective tissue. The antibody and antigen react, causing the mast cells to react and release chemicals, including histamine.[5] Antibodies are specific to antigens, so, for example, antibodies to cows' milk may exist in the gut and nose, while antibodies to pollen may only exist in the nose and throat—which helps to explain why different areas are sometimes affected by different allergens.

Food for thought

TWO TYPES OF IMMUNE REACTION

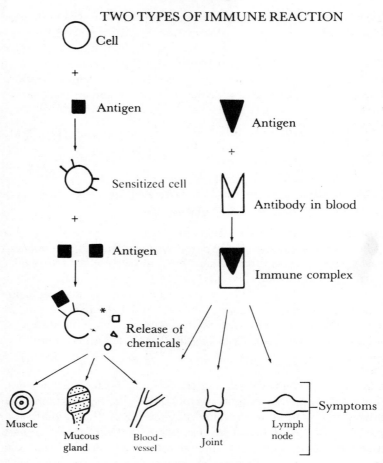

Fig. 1.1. What happens in allergic reactions.

Some antigens reach the body's mucous surfaces, and then penetrate into the bloodstream, where they may be carried around the body, causing symptoms in any number of internal organs. Of these antigens, some may attach themselves to red blood cells, some to platelets, and some to white blood cells. Others come into contact with specific antibodies in the blood, and lock together to form immune complexes. These immune complexes may be stationary or circulating, causing direct tissue injury or causing other reactions which produce injury. The injury will vary with the kind of cell involved, quantity of antigen, etc. Often, of course, different reactions are taking place simultaneously. But the type III reaction is worth describing more fully—'The antigen and antibody react together in tissue spaces, and a precipitate is formed which can block small blood-vessels. It takes several hours to start after exposure to the offending antigen, and may last from 24 to 36 hours. The reaction may include a fever, pains in the muscles, aching, and a rise in the number of white cells in the blood.'[6] This sounds suspiciously like the limb and joint pains that trouble otherwise healthy children at night, in many cases, always after eating a particular food or foods. Philip, the first case history, is a good example of this reaction. The pain may vary from moderate to excruciating—it caused him to be hospitalized at the age of three.

That, very roughly, is *allergy*. However, just to make things more difficult, some specialists consider only type I reactions to be 'allergy' even though historically this is not the definition.

WHAT HAPPENS IN INTOLERANT REACTIONS?

What of non-immunological adverse reactions, variously called intolerance, hypersensitivity, or idiosyncrasy? The symptoms produced may be identical to those produced by allergy. What is different is simply *how* they are produced. Because the body is so complex, there are any number of biochemical mistakes or anomalies that can cause problems. One example: the body may be deficient in, or lacking, a specific enzyme needed to digest a certain food. This deficiency or lack may be permanent or temporary, inherited or acquired. A simple example would be the disease state known as PKU (phenylketonuria). The PKU infant lacks the genes for the enzyme needed to breakdown phenylalanine. Without it, this substance will go on building up in the bloodstream and damage sensitive tissues like the brain.

But the causes of disease states are rarely so simple. Let's look at lactose intolerance, for example.[8] This comes about when the body cannot tolerate lactose, one of the sugars present in varying amounts in mammalian milks, because it has insufficient lactase, the enzyme needed to break down lactose. The sugar therefore reaches the intestines, where it 'draws out water from the gut walls

Food for thought

by osmosis, and is fermented. The result is highly acid, profuse watery diarrhoea and crampy bowel spasms. If diarrhoea is prolonged, the gut is further damaged by the acid, and may not be able to digest other foods due to further loss of other enzymes, etc. The loss of the protective coating of immunoglobulin A may also allow secondary food intolerances to develop, which then prolongs the diarrhoea and results in permanent allergy to cows' milk, or whatever other food was present in some quantity while the gut lining was damaged. This has practical implications for the feeding of children with diarrhoea, obviously.

Unlike PKU, however, lactose intolerance is only rarely an inborn problem. Human milk the world over is uniformly high in lactose, and almost no baby is born unable to cope with lactose, even though there is wide variance in inborn levels of lactase. How and why does lactose intolerance develop? Why is it so commonly diagnosed in Australia, where, unlike the majority of the world's tribes and races, the majority of Caucasian Australian adults will produce the enzyme lactase? Could it be that this apparent epidemic of lactose intolerance in babies is due to avoidable factors such as:

(a) Early sensitization to cows' milk because of the once almost universal practice of complementary feeds in hospital; and the continued reaction to cows' milk in the breast-feeding mother's diet. (Australian mothers consume quite excessive quantities of dairy products, sometimes on medical advice.)[9]
(b) The dramatic persistent changes to infant gut flora brought about by even one feed of animal milks or solid foods.[10]
(c) A deficiency of protective substances in maternal milk, e.g. mild iron deficiency causes a decrease in antibody formation.
(d) An oversupply of toxins such as nicotine or any of the other thousands of chemicals in cigarette smoke; environmental contaminants of all kinds.
(e) For the bottle-fed infant, deficiency in particular amino acids, trace elements or vitamins, which, even if present in some formulae,[11] are not so well absorbed in the absence of the carrier proteins found in human milk, and in the presence of pathogenic (disease-causing) bacteria.
(f) The unique Western cultural habit of giving babies big feeds at intervals of 3–4 hours, rather than smaller, more

8

frequent feeds. The newborn is not designed for such alternating periods of overfeeding and starvation.[12]

Of course, there are two other possibilities:

(1) That lactose intolerance is readily diagnosed because a cheap, simple test for it exists. The test, however, is simply a crude measure of how much lactose is in a baby's stools. Lactose is greatly reduced in a bottle-fed baby's stools because of the unnaturally delayed transit time of his food; no-one seems to have stated what the normal range of lactose is for the breast-fed baby's stools. Yet breast-fed babies who are cheerful, and not losing weight, are sometimes taken from the breast because the Clinitest reading exceeds 0.5 per cent. Prominent gastroenterologists and paediatricians deplore this use of the test. In one major hospital, children with 2 per cent lactose will be breast-fed for as long as their clinical signs show they are not deteriorating.

(2) That lactose intolerance is a symptom, not a cause, i.e. that it happens secondary to the effect on the gut lining of some other excitant. Lactose intolerance may develop after cows' milk intolerance, for example. This explains why some babies do very badly on lactose-free formulae made from cows' milk protein, and also why lactose intolerance can be persistent or recurring in a breast-fed baby whose mother does not alter her own diet to avoid likely allergens.

I have not been able to determine whether lactose intolerance is diagnosed as readily, and managed as badly, in the UK as in Australia. Readers might like to tell me of their experiences with this problem. Obviously those of Asian and African origins will have more problems as adults should they persist in drinking milk, but I am especially interested in childhood lactose intolerance.

The relationships between nutrition and disease are extremely varied and complex, and only just beginning to be researched. For some excellent recent studies, I would recommend the series being published by Plenum Press—*Human nutrition, A comprehensive treatise* (ed. Winick); Lebenthal's *Textbook of gastroenterology and nutrition in infancy*; the Jelliffe's *Adverse effects of foods*; Lessof's *Clinical reactions to food*; Soothill *et al. Paediatric immunology*; and Wilkinson's, *The immunology of infant feeding*. (See the Bibliography pp. 213–33).

2

Effects and victims of food intolerance

HOW DO THESE PROBLEMS INTERRELATE?

Biochemical anomalies are not only inherited, however. They may also be the result of other bodily malfunctioning, as the Fig. 2.1 illustrates. For millions of children, malnutrition is the point of entry into the vicious cycle described. In 'developed' countries, the point of entry is quite possibly related to our radical, new, untested, and inappropriate infant-feeding practices. And I want to emphasize that although such practices as bottle-feeding may *seem* culturally normal, they are experiments with human infants which could not now be introduced without rigorous and careful testing. That testing was never done. Yet there are even academics who argue that we should 'prove' breast-feeding to be superior.[1] Who proved bottle-feeding was ever even adequate, much less superior, before launching massive advertising campaigns?

Malnutrition does not only mean an absolute lack of food. It also means a lack of the right foods for one's particular needs.[2] A deficiency of even one essential amino acid, or vitamin, or trace element, or mineral may substantially alter the body's capacity to handle other foods and to grow properly.

Infection, too, can be the starting-point for entry into this vicious cycle. The baby who is not being exclusively breast-fed has many harmful bacteria flourishing in his bowel. He is much more vulnerable to bacterial or viral invaders, and almost certainly will have more episodes of gastroenteritis, ear infections, and so on. Infection increases the body's need for nutrients to combat the invaders, and almost always results in changes in appetite and growth. If certain types of bacteria are involved, the toxins they produce in the gut will damage it, making it easier for the child to be sensitized to foods and causing diarrhoea (see Fig. 2.1). If the child is given antibiotics, these too have an impact (cf. p. 12).

Infection may mean things other than bacteria and viruses. We can also be infected with fungi such as candida (thrush), protozoa such as malaria and giardia, and worms of various sorts. All of

10

Effects and victims of food intolerance

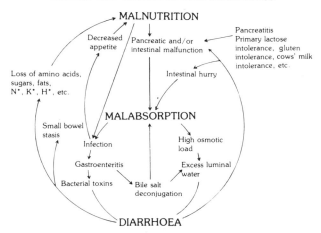

Fig. 1.2. The vicious cycle of diarrhoea and malnutrition.

these organisms have an impact on how well the gut handles food, affecting both the absorption of nutrients, the levels of enzymes, and the health of the gut mucosa.[3] A child with worms is not uncommon, and not serious. An allergic child with worms may be at greater risk of further sensitization to new foods or drugs taken if his gut lining has been damaged. So it is worth watching for the tell-tale signs: night restlesness, itchy bottom, etc. However, here again the allergic child may have problems: the most effective worm medicines come in highly coloured and flavoured forms, and the worm remedy may cause yet another problem. Hence it is sensible to be sure of the diagnosis. Once the child has been asleep and is warm, take a torch and check the anus during a bout of restlessness. If you see fine threads moving, give the whole family a dose and follow all the disinfection procedures—change beds and clothes, cut and scrub fingernails, etc.[4]

Giardia is now being recognized as a common intestinal parasite, more difficult to detect than worms, but associated with chronic or intermittent diarrhoea.[5] Once again, both disease and treatment pose problems for the allergic child, so it is as well to be sure of the diagnosis. Many mothers reported that a child prescribed 'Flagyl' for giardia reacted badly to the drug–cf. case history 6. Human milk has recently been shown to kill giardia.[6]

Food for thought

Though it is not yet clear whether this would be completely effective in all breast-fed babies, there is certainly no case for weaning when the mother has giardia.

Overgrowths of thrush can also be associated with bowel problems,[7] just as overgrowths of gut bacteria can be. The difficulty in both of these is re-establishing the normal balance of the gut flora. That balance can be disrupted by broad-spectrum antibiotics— which wipe out useful as well as harmful bacteria and so allow non-affected organisms to grow unchecked. It can also be disrupted by unbalanced diets—thrush is said to thrive on a sugar-rich diet, for example. Several people mentioned that gut disturbances were improved by the use of anti-fungal medication, yoghurt, or special capsules containing useful bacteria such as lactobacillus. Here your doctor or chemist could help—but remember to check the ingredients if you are food-intolerant!

All along I have stated that these infections are associated with gut problems. There is a chicken and egg problem here. Which comes first? Do these people become infected because an underlying problem such as food intolerance predisposes them to, or because their resistance is lower than other people's? Or does the infection produce secondary food intolerances? Why is it that one child goes to school and in his first year catches everything, while a second child in the same group stays well all year? It is not simply that one child is exposed and the other not exposed—we are constantly exposed to all manner of infective agents. The basis must be the difference in the efficiency of one child's immune system—and that, as we have said earlier, is the result of a very complicated interaction between heredity, environment, nutrition, and the rest. So don't look for easy answers. If the doctor says 'It's giardia', without any tests to ascertain it, he may or may not be right. Even if he is right, that doesn't end the matter. Is giardia also a symptom, of some immune deficiency perhaps? Or secondary to food intolerance? None of these answers is sufficient by itself, and only time and careful observation will tell you the most likely solution in an individual case.

Teething, oddly enough, may also fit in here. I'm told that teething alters the relative acidity of saliva and that this in turn alters digestion. (Some breast-feeding mothers find that their nipples become sore and are eased by bathing with a mild solution of bicarbonate of soda—a teaspoon to a pint of water or so.) Cer-

Effects and victims of food intolerance

tainly teething is a stress for many babies—the inflammation of the gums, and pain, are obvious. This would cause stress hormones to be released, and so affect bodily functioning, including the handling of antigens. Teething plus immunization is a disastrous combination for some babies. Which is not an argument against immunization, but a request for thorough investigation of the most appropriate time for immunization of allergic and high-risk infants.

WHO IS AT RISK IN DEVELOPED COUNTRIES?

It is easy to see that a hungry Third World child is at risk,[8] but less obvious risks exist in affluent countries, and too many of our children are needlessly exposed to them.

The newborn baby is at particular risk. Both his immunological and digestive systems are immature. He relies upon immunoglobulins and other substances in his mother's milk to protect him until his immune system is fully functioning.[9] That milk is uniquely digestible because it contains nutrients in exactly the right amounts and composition as well as many enzymes[10] that the baby lacks, and special 'carrier proteins' which enable the body to utilize the nutrients while preventing them from being available to the gut bacteria. (This influences the type and growth of bacteria present.) So human milk for the human infant provides food, some of the enzymes needed to digest it, and a variety of substances which provide protection against infection. In addition, one specific immunoglobulin, IgA, acts as a 'paint', coating the infant intestine, reducing absorption of, and the risk of sensitization to, any foreign protein. For the newborn intestinal lining is relatively permeable, allowing quite large molecules to pass into the blood.[11] If the child is exposed to a potential allergen at this time,[12] he is far more likely to be sensitized. Note here that we are not necessarily trying to prevent a child from being exposed at all to food antigens. From recent research in Perth, it seems that tolerance (the ability to handle antigens correctly) may be induced by exposing the infant upper respiratory tract to quantities of antigen sufficient to both switch on an immune response, and more importantly, to switch it off again before symptoms develop.[13] This means that both the presence of antigen in mothers' milk (which seems to be almost universal) and the style of feeding (breast milk being forcibly ejected from the breast in a spray, unlike its slow extraction from a bottle) are possibly beneficial, increasing the likelihood of tolerance being induced. One of the principal researchers involved acknowledges that there is likely to be significant inhalation of breast milk, whereas it is widely recognized that inhalation of foreign milks is a considerable hazard. (Inhalation of other species' milk induced anaphylaxis and death in guinea pigs; mothers' milk had no effect whatever.) Whatever the role of upper respiratory or gastrointestinal tracts, there seems likely to be good reason to prefer breast milk.

Tolerance or sensitivity may be induced in various ways. One route consistently neglected by many researchers is that of intra-uterine exposure. This is despite the fact that it is known that sensitisation can occur *in utero*, especially when mothers eat some foods in excess. It would seem that if a mother-to-be or lactating mother 'binges' on highly allergenic food such as milk, cheese, chocolate, citrus fruits, or eggs, in pregnancy[13] or lactation, very high levels of that potential allergen may be circulating in her milk or blood. Even higher levels will probably be circulating if she happens to be in a state of active allergy, with her own gut abnormally permeable to excitants and antigens. In highly allergic (atopic) families, that could certainly be enough to sensitize the baby. (There is evidence of less than normal immunoglobulin (Ig) production in atopic families, so that quantities harmless to others cannot be coped with.) It is quite possible that human milk is designed to expose a baby to tiny quantities of the normal foods of that culture, so that he can cope with weaning. Binges by a mother with a damaged gut lining (perhaps the long-term results of *her* early childhood diet?) may provide enough antigen to sensitize the child *in utero* or via her milk.

The problem might not necessarily be with the absolute amount of antigen circulating in the mother's bloodstream, but in the baby's response to that amount. Studies on breast-feeding mothers of babies with and without eczema reveal widely differing amounts of common antigens, but there was not a perfect correspondence between high levels and symptoms. Perhaps it depended on combinations of antigens, on prostaglandin levels, on inbuilt defects in the baby's immune system, or on amount, type, and site of initial exposure—the variables are many. Until it is possible to elucidate all relevant mechanisms in individual cases, we are left

14

with more questions than answers. Yet as guidelines for managing such infants we must adopt those procedures that do as little harm to physiological systems as possible.

A great deal of evidence suggests that this must mean the end of practices such as hospital feeding of formulae to newborns. It is clear that the early introduction of foreign foods is harmful to children of atopic families and of many 'normal' families, as well as to every other young mammal ever studied. It greatly increases the chances of sensitization for even the least atopic family.[15] In the mid-1970s, fewer than 14 per cent of all children born in hospitals in the UK escaped being given complementary feeds of cows' milk formulae.[15] This practice, from being uncommon and expensive, became almost universal in some hospitals after companies made supplies available to hospitals at little or no cost. Of course such feedings interfere with the successful establishment of breast-feeding,[16] and are almost totally unnecessary where midwives and doctors are properly educated about the management of lactation.[17] Fortunately the practice seems to be disappearing rapidly as its serious risks become recognized. Unfortunately, no concerted effort to re-educate nursing staff has taken place in some areas, and the result is that while a hospital may have a policy of 'no comps', a casual night sister, trained in the bottle's heyday, may revert to doing what she thinks is best, sometimes without even recording the fact. Many mothers have been shocked to discover that the baby who 'slept through, Mrs Jones', had in fact been given two or more bottles that night. Australia's freedom of information legislation has made such discoveries possible about past births, though it may lead to changes in what is recorded now that staff know that parents can gain access to records. Parents who are in any doubt about their child's feeding ought to write to the hospital concerned and request full details, while remaining aware that all records are fallible. (Organizations such as are listed in the Resources section (p. 191) will help you discover your rights in dealing with hospitals.)

But if the practice of giving complementary feeds is so risky, why don't *all* exposed children manifest symptoms? It is just possible that in fact almost all do, in varying degrees. But before we look at the question, let us consider the question of symptoms.

3

General symptoms

Symptoms should be seen as the tip of the iceberg. Human bodies are remarkably adaptable, and have many sophisticated mechanisms for coping with challenges of all kinds. Whether or not a particular challenge results in *what are recognized as clinical symptoms* seems to depend on the balance between the body's total load and its current tolerance level, threshold, or ceiling,[1] The following diagrams, reproduced with permission from Professor Rapp, will illustrate this.

TOTAL BODY LOAD AND CURRENT TOLERANCE LEVEL

The total body load comprises the amount of every antigen or excitant that the body is presently exposed to—in one case perhaps milk, cat hair, and pollen, although there are usually many. (Inhalant allergies may take weeks or years to develop; infant sneezing is often a response to a dietary or viral allergen.) At certain times and in certain amounts these produce no symptoms, as the body's current tolerance ceiling varies too. Additional stress—fatigue, poor nutrition, cold, emotional strain, infection, drugs—will lower its current tolerance level so that food which caused no symptoms last week may produce symptoms this week. ('Because' it turned cold, or 'because' the rye grass is flowering, or 'because' you changed the beds, or 'because' you had an argument, and so on, allergic reactions are triggered off.) This is now clearly recognized as occurring in both animals and man. As the Joint Report of the Royal College of Physicians and British Nutrition Foundation (hereafter the RCP/BNF Report) stated, immune reactions to food 'can be produced in experimental animals either spontaneously [following regular feeding of antigen] or by manipulating the immune status of an animal, or its environment, at

16

General symptoms

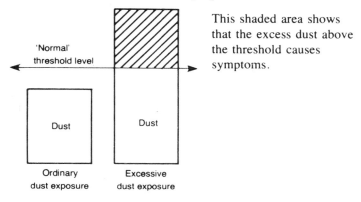

This shaded area shows that the excess dust above the threshold causes symptoms.

This shows how a child who is allergic to dust has no symptoms when the total dust exposure is below the child's threshold for symptoms.

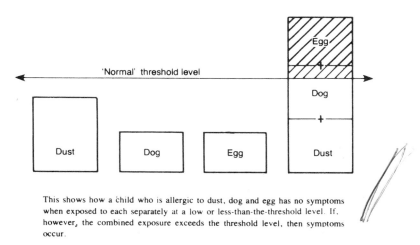

This shows how a child who is allergic to dust, dog and egg has no symptoms when exposed to each separately at a low or less-than-the-threshold level. If, however, the combined exposure exceeds the threshold level, then symptoms occur.

Fig. 3.1. Examples of allergy thresholds. (From Rapp, D. (1980), *Allergies and your family*. Sterling Publishing Co., New York.)

the time of antigen feeding.'[2] This could be done by, for example, giving antigen and whooping cough adjuvant. In people, it has since been shown that what was thought to be exercise-induced anaphylaxis is food-dependent[3] and that without the food having been eaten, exercise did not cause distress. In such cases, the food

17

Food for thought

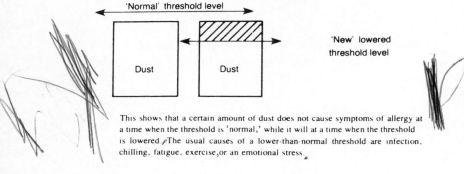

'Normal' threshold level

'New' lowered threshold level

Dust

Dust

This shows that a certain amount of dust does not cause symptoms of allergy at a time when the threshold is 'normal,' while it will at a time when the threshold is lowered. The usual causes of a lower-than-normal threshold are infection, chilling, fatigue, exercise, or an emotional stress.

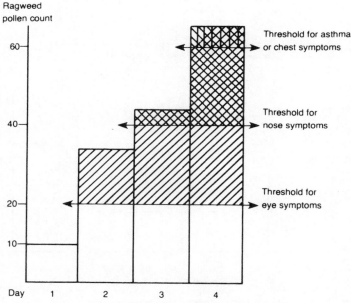

Ragweed pollen count

Threshold for asthma or chest symptoms

Threshold for nose symptoms

Threshold for eye symptoms

Day

This diagram shows how a child who is allergic to ragweed has no symptoms when the ragweed count is below 20, has eye symptoms when it is above 20, eye and nose symptoms when it is above 40, and eye, nose, and chest (asthma) symptoms when the count is over 60.

Fig. 3.2. Examples of allergy thresholds. (From Rapp,. D. (1980), *Allergies and your family*, Sterling Publishing Co., New York.)

18

must be seen as the underlying cause, and exercise simply as the trigger for symptoms. Another recent study showed that someone who could normally eat peanuts without any adverse effects suffered from anaphylaxis on one occasion when he did so. It turned out that he had also ingested aspirin a short time beforehand.[4] The aspirin had apparently potentiated the reaction in some way—but peanuts were the cause. Convincing such people that foods they sometimes eat without effect may cause occasional problems, depending on other interacting factors, can be very difficult. Convincing someone else can be impossible. It should be easier now that the RCP/BNF Report has stated that, 'even in sensitive subjects, the response [to challenges] . . . is inconsistent and may occur only in the presence of potentiating factors.[5]

The child who can eat milk on his cereal at weekends without trouble may *genuinely* experience stomach pains on school days because of the additional stress or different chemicals, dust, etc. involved in school life. Bowel and bladder control can vary in similar ways. Toilet training can be very difficult; the toilet-trained child may have inexplicable accidents; bed-wetting is common. All the above emphasizes the urgency of identifying as many of the family's allergies and intolerances as possible: not necessarily so that they can be avoided totally—that may not prove essential—but so that at times of greater stress parents know which small manipulations of diet or contact may bring the child's total load down below his symptom threshold, and, even more importantly, so that parents do not get involved in dreadful battles with a child over behaviour that he is *not* responsible for. Night waking, difficult toilet training, terrible tantrums, poor concentration, hyperactivity, and a host of awful behaviours can be the result of the biochemical effects of certain foods.[6] (Not always, of course, and behaviour once learnt becomes habitual in families, but there have been dramatic unexpected improvements both in parents and in children.)

The body's current tolerance level normally rises as the child grows. Around two it reaches a plateau which often means that eczema lessens or disappears and some forms of aggressive behaviour change. (The decrease in milk intake at 1–2 could be significant for many babies too.) Asthma may suddenly emerge—no-one knows why, though it could be related to increased social stress—around 4–5, although many children

19

develop asthma much younger. Around 8–10 years another postulated improvement in immune functioning sometimes 'causes' asthma to lessen or disappear. However, here too other factors may be just as important. No mother 'pushes' milk or eggs to a 10-year-old as she does to a pre-schooler; by that age the child's wishes are sometimes taken more seriously. It is never safe to assert that the cause of such changes is known with certainty[3]—the child is changing but so is his environment.[7]

IS ONE CURED WHEN SYMPTOM-FREE?

Probably not.[8] Primed antibodies may continue to exist within the body just as they do for bacterial invaders. There are two common mistakes made here:

1. Parents assume that when, for example, eczema or asthma disappear, the child is cured. When they reintroduce foods without provoking either eczema or asthma, they are sure of it. When the child complains of headache, has nose bleeds, or joint pains, they assume that these are 'normal' rather than possibly indicating continued intolerance manifest in different target organs.

2. Parents assume that it is 'better' for the child to learn to cope with some of the foods to which he is intolerant—socially more acceptable, and perhaps even physically less dangerous.

Here it is simply not clear whether or not parents are right. The child may be experiencing symptoms which are not recognized as such—behavioural effects, for example, or inflammation of bladder or pancreas or other glands. He *may* be coping with these problems without any internal effects. But if his immune system is coping with food antigens, is it more or less capable of dealing with infective organisms? If the child has what is regarded as the 'normal' number of colds, earaches, tonsillitis, or whatever (including in little girls, vulvo-vaginitis and cystitis), then I believe that complete avoidance of known antigens is definitely called for. Of course, this implies that you have other good reasons for suspecting allergy and have in fact identified food allergens. This has been criticized publicly[9] by an immunologist as sounding as though all children who have eight or nine colds annually ought to be off milk

Food for thought

and other foods year round. I hope you will read the book carefully enough to see that I am not advocating any such blanket approach. The fact is however that hundreds of parents are now aware that the 'normal' number of colds is no longer normal for their children. Not a few ear, nose, and throat specialists have reached the same conclusion about themselves and their patients. Case history 5 (p. 182) illustrates this point very nicely.

Our cultural conceptions about what constitutes normal good health have probably been subtly shaped by the ever increasing incidence of allergic disease[10] in this society. We need to keep an historical and cultural perspective on such issues.

ABOUT ADAPTATION AND ADDICTION

Another reason for symptoms disappearing can be that the person has become adapted to his antigens. He feels normal only while he has his regular 'fix' of milk, or coffee, tea, or tomatoes. Going without causes withdrawal symptoms every bit as unpleasant as the non-addicted allergic suffers on exposure to the same food. This is common in the toddler, who often, after vomiting milk for some months, suddenly develops a passion for it and 'lives on it'—no other food is acceptable. At the same time his behaviour often worsens,[11] but we accept that the 'terrible two's' are a normal stage of development, and the mother is counselled to accept him as he is. Similarly, it is not uncommon for his mother to be unable to get through a day with such a child without innumerable cups of tea or coffee, or cigarettes; her mental confusion and difficulty in remembering much without lists is put down to the pressures and distractions of living with children. In at least some cases both mother and child change dramatically if they can survive the withdrawal period.

Eventually the strain on the body (which involves mobilization of hormones, etc.) may become too great, and severe symptoms become evident. Recovery is more difficult because of the effects on the endocrine (hormone-producing) glands. But at this stage it is once again clear that the former addictant now produces illness. This theory was first formulated by Professor Hans Selye, of the University of Montreal, one of the world's foremost authorities on stress and the diseases of adaptation. It is well set out by Mackarness[12] from whence Fig. 3.3 comes.

21

Food for thought

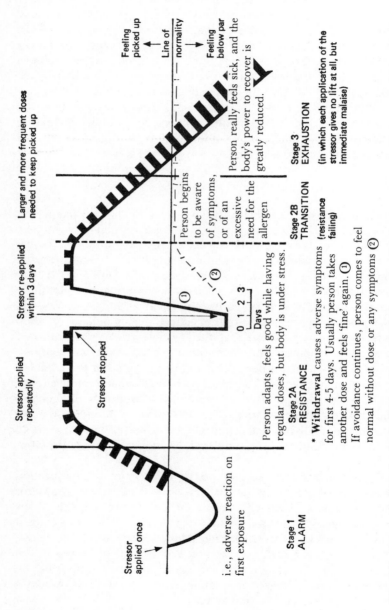

Fig. 3.3. Stages of adaptation and addition. (Adapted from Mackarness, R. (1980) *Chemical victims*, Pan Books London.)

General symptoms

On the other hand, although there is little scientific evidence to support this, some parents who continually expose their children to minute amounts of a food that they are intolerant of have reported that in time even normal amounts seem to cause no problems. The original sensitivity seems to have been overcome, or at least to have altered.

What is one to make of this? It could simply be an unrecognized state of adaptation. But it could possibly work—after all, this could be how a 'normal' baby develops tolerance of foods eaten by his non-allergic mother: constant exposure to the tiny amounts in human milk. Desensitization by injection is thought to work for inhalant allergies, though there is some debate about the safety of such procedures in certain cases, and such injections during pregnancy have been associated by some parents with abnormally intolerant babies. However, American and Canadian allergists insist that treatment during pregnancy is positively beneficial to the child, stimulating immunity to the allergens. This may prove to be an individual matter. But as sudden rises in body temperature have been shown to be potentially harmful to infants *in utero*, any mother who reacts to injections with a fever ought definitely to avoid them in pregnancy. I personally would err on the side of caution and avoid any such sudden stimulus to the immune system.

So once again, we do not really know. Advocates of this theory stress that it must be constant, graduated exposure—no stops and starts. This may be as much bother as avoidance of the allergen. There is one practical point: this might suggest that pregnant and lactating women ought to avoid only those foods which cause definite symptoms, and ought to eat all other foods constantly in moderation.[13] It may be the constant monotony of diet in 'peasant' cultures which induces infant tolerance. Perhaps choice and variety and so a wide variation in intake, is why affluence and allergy are associated? Once again, no one seems to have studied this. And as we will discuss later, there is constant debate within the medical profession over the question of whether large or small amounts are more or less likely to lead to tolerance. You will be sadly disillusioned if you think the experts know it all—their own clinical experience, that is what they do to patients, proceeds not from 'scientific proof' but from experimentation, hypothesis, and the odd dash of prejudice in some cases!

Food for thought

CAN SYMPTOMS RETURN?

Obviously yes, if adaptation fails. But new symptoms can develop at literally any time of life. Periods of great physical or emotional stress may precipitate them. Before exams, a wedding, pregnancy (especially when one has other young children), childbirth, marital discord, job changes, moving house—all may so lower one's threshold that symptoms develop. Obviously it is a good idea to keep records of problems in childhood—it could save a great deal of family strain if known excitants are avoided at times of predictable stress. Furthermore, intolerant girl children could grow up to produce babies sensitized *in utero* unless they take special care. (I have been astonished at how often mothers reported that after consulting their parents they found positive evidence of their own inability to tolerate cows' milk in infancy. Many were brought up on goats' milk and other products; many had eczema, hives, or asthma; many loathed milk and were sick every day after drinking the compulsory school milk, or had 'notes' to avoid it.) And with a greater appreciation of the impact of 'minor' dietary deficiency—such as zinc or some trace elements—parents probably need to take care to educate all their children in the importance of good diet, and the subtle effects of minor malabsorption, which is especially likely in food-intolerant patients because of the effect on the gut lining.[14] (This will of course be regarded as nonsense or neurosis by those who know very little about nutrition, but there is fascinating research connecting inadequate diet and problems of fertility, congenital defects, stillbirths and mental defect.)[15] Any UK reader interested in this should contact Foresight (see p. 195).

CAN A PERSON BECOME ALLERGIC LATER IN LIFE?

Yes, 'Allergic breakthrough' is particularly likely after gastroenteritis or diarrhoea, when the gut has not yet recovered.[16] It is possible at any time that the body is exposed to massive amounts of any one substance and the body's resistance is low. Perhaps it happens less often because adult diet is generally more varied. There is no pressure to, for example, eat more than one eighth of one's total body weight of one food—which the *bottle-fed* baby does daily. 'Binges' of any food are thus best avoided. Here it is interesting to note that some alcoholics are thought to be allergic to the grains or yeasts of their favourite drinks. They are in the addicted stage, so that withdrawal caused symptoms and exposure a return to normalcy[17] (see p. 21). Some were said to be unable to cure the alcohol addiction until they had identified and eliminated the grains in normal food forms, to which they were sensitive. That does not mean that all those with a drink problem ought to drop cereals from their diet—the alcoholic more than most needs an excellent diet and nutritional counselling. But there are people working in drug and alcohol referral centres who could help. It is also interesting to notice how many former alcoholics seem to crave sugar, caffeine, and nicotine—or socially acceptable drugs. Apparent allergic breakthrough is also reported in older women, where marked hormonal changes have occurred.[16]

There is no such thing as a 'non-allergic' person. Although only about 10% of people manifest major allergy . . . and 50% of people manifest either major or minor allergy, some time in their lives, these manifestations can come on at any age. Since my child is potentially allergic, it is intelligent to protect him from unnecessary risks which may bring on serious and perhaps prolonged allergic symptoms and even disability.

Cecil Collins Williams, *Paediatric allergy and clinical immunology* p. 82. Churchill Livingstone (1973).

4

Food intolerance in infancy

COMMON SYMPTOMS IN INFANCY

The argument runs that cows' milk given to infants has been proved safe because many 'comp'-ed breast-fed babies and bottle-fed infants are not significantly different in health or behaviour.[1] There are obvious fallacies in this reasoning; nor is it accurate in the light of recent studies, which show a clear connection between feeding and incidence and severity of illness.[2] This will be one of the topics I hope to go into at some length in a book on infant feeding. However, once again I would stress the massive scale of commerciogenic, or profit-motivated, dietary changes in our society in the last century. Such massive changes could be expected to create a new cultural stereotype of what is 'normal' health and behaviour. Important medical discoveries such as antibiotics may well have served to camouflage the impact of these radical, uncontrolled changes. We in the West regard infant crying as normal, and in a thousand different ways condition our children to associate babies with bawling.[3] But in societies where infants are exclusively breast-fed from birth and in contact with their non-allergic, non-food-bingeing, non-smoking mothers, 'colic' is unknown and infant crying is seen as a sign of distress, which warrants immediate attention.[4] And that is exactly what it sounds like to the new mother, until she is persuaded by others, against every instinct she possesses, that this is 'normal' or 'naughty', depending on her social background, and must be treated with drugs or punishment, or both.

IS COLIC FOOD-RELATED?

The definition of colic is to some extent subjective. Which is not surprising, since babies and parents are individuals and have widely differing pain/inconvenience thresholds, as well as widely differing expectations of life. It is probably pointless to try to quantify and define how much and what sort of crying constitutes

26

colic. For our purposes, a colicky baby is one that screams or cries enough to distress its parents, sleeps little or restlessly, and who gives the impression of having sometimes intense abdominal pain. The breast-fed colicky baby usually feeds, or suckles, as often as he can, for the breast provides solace. However, he may also begin to suckle, then pull away and cry desperately after a few minutes. These babies are healthy, usually gaining weight adequately (sometimes, but not always, despite very frequent stools), and have been checked by the doctor for other problems such as gastro-oesophageal reflux.

Only a few years ago, to suggest that such babies could be food intolerant was to invite medical ridicule by experts. Today, you will be pleased to know, most of the experts—but not all, of course—agree that colicky babies may be food-intolerant. The real question for the academic is now not 'whether', but 'how many?'[5] A rather disturbing indication emerges from a study of colicky bottle-fed infants. The babies were changed to soy formulae—only 18 per cent improved. Another 53 per cent improved on formulae such as Pregestimil and Nutramigen although some later proved to be intolerant even of those. In short, at least 71 per cent of those colicky bottle-fed babies were milk intolerant and many were intolerant of more than one type of formula.[6] For more on this, see p. 120.

Wider acceptance of the link between colic and food intolerance may be hampered by the Joint Report of the Royal College of Physicians and British Nutrition Foundation, *Food intolerance and food aversion* (referred to as the RCP/BNF Report). Apropos of colic, the report acknowledges that, 'It is striking how many infants . . . subsequently shown to have cows' milk protein intolerance have in the past had persistent screaming and colic.' So far so good. But it goes on to say that, 'Withdrawal of cows' milk from the diet of breast-feeding mothers was shown to be followed by improvement in colic in an uncontrolled study, but not in a subsequent controlled trial. The association between infantile colic and food intolerance thus remains to be proven, but may well be significant in those in whom overt atopic symptoms subsequently develop.[7]

How fair a summary of the research is this? And should we wait until colicky babies become asthmatics before suspecting food intolerance?

Food for thought

The uncontrolled study referred to was the original 1978 study by Jakobsson and Lindberg.[8] Since then they have published a prospective study of cows' milk protein intolerance, showing colic as a symptom;[9] the double blind study of colicky bottle-fed infants referred to earlier, showing a staggering rate of food intolerance;[10] and a double-blind cross-over study of breast-fed infants, which showed that many babies improved when cows' milk was eliminated from their mothers' diets.[11] Further corroboration came from Canada,[12] and from the UK itself.[13] None of these are cited in the RCP/BNF Report. Instead, we are referred to a subsequent 'controlled trial' which was thought to contradict their results. This New Zealand study[14] has received world-wide publicity. What exactly was done, and what can be safely concluded from it?

Over one 12-day period, 20 New Zealand mothers were told to go on a milk-free diet. Every day each mother was given a 600 ml drink to swallow before noon; in alternating two-day blocks this was either 600 ml Isomil (soy milk) plus flavouring, *or* 300 ml Isomil + 300 ml cows' milk plus flavouring. There was no significant difference in the baby's colic on soy-only days as compared with soy + milk days. The researchers also noted that colic increased steadily as mothers ate more of a selection of common allergens—milk, eggs, chocolate, fruit, nuts, fish. Their conclusion was that 'maternal diet may influence the likelihood of infantile colic in breastfed children, but that the source of the colic cannot be attributed to a single dietary component. It may, however, involve a variety of foodstuffs.'

No doubt the Swedish researchers, Jakobsson and Lindberg, would agree and this is also clearly our Australian experience. The logical next step is to discover ways of determining which foods affect which babies, and why. But did this study really exonerate cows' milk as the most likely cause of infantile colic in infants commonly given formula in hospital and breast-fed by mothers drinking litres of milk? Hardly. The defects in the methodology of this study should be obvious to anyone.

Consider the following points:

— Intervals between challenges were two or four days, yet intervals of up to two weeks may be needed for symptoms of previous reactions to subside (see p. 148.)
— Milk is used as a beverage. No mention is made of what

28

mothers drank instead of milk. Did they drink more tea, coffee, orange juice, or other potential allergens? What other dietary changes were made?

— Avoiding hidden milk is extremely difficult. How complete was the mothers' avoidance of milk protein?

— 300 ml of cows' milk is a small amount if the mothers are used to consuming litres. What was the normal dietary intake of bovine protein, and what would be the result of challenging mothers with *that* amount?

— Soy products are unusual in the New Zealand diet. 600 ml Isomil is thus a large amount of an uncommon, high sugar, and notoriously 'windy' food for adults not used to it. Is this a suitable 'control'?

— Alternatively, if soy milks contain essential fatty acids likely to help control symptoms (see pp. 47, 238–9), will some mothers and babies be helped by this, while others without nutritional problems react adversely?

— How much flavouring was there, and how inert was it?

What this study did was to compare the colic-inducing capacity of a small amount of a common allergen plus a relatively large amount of an uncommon allergen (300 ml milk + 300 ml soy) with the colic-inducing capacity of a large amount of one uncommon allergen (600 ml soy)—plus various other changes in diet, untabulated. These mothers may have rearranged some components of their total allergen load, but they were certainly not identifying and avoiding their allergens. The only meaningful comparisons are those between mothers consuming normal (that is, normal for them) amounts of cows' milk, and those not consuming any, and not altering their diet in other ways, over a period of at least two weeks. Some may improve in a few days, but others will not. Since cows' milk may not be the most important allergen in some cases, one need not rule out food intolerance if this still shows no result. Indeed, I never begin with milk unless there is reason to suspect it (see p. 143).

So we really do not know whether this handful of New Zealand mothers had problems with milk, with Isomil, with neither, or both. What we do know is that as they ate more of Western society's most common allergens, the babies' colic increased. Could a follow-up study be done, to see whether those children now react

Food for thought

to milk, to the ingredients of Isomil as it was then formulated, or to other foods? How many are not atopic?

It is extraordinary that this study, with its clear support for a link between maternal diet and infant colic, could be used to support any statement that this link 'remains to be proven'. Where is the contradiction between the Swedes' and others finding cows' milk to be a major dietary allergen and the New Zealanders' finding that many foods can cause colic? Australian mothers agree with both. The question researchers need to tackle is not *whether* colic can be food-related, but how to identify those foods that are, and to explain why this person, why this food, and why these symptoms.

It also seems extraordinary to me that the other studies have been overlooked. There is naturally a reluctance to accept findings which implicitly raise doubts as to the wisdom of past procedures once accepted as safe, such as early formula feeding; or which cast doubts upon cherished theories of infant crying being due to inadequate mothers. But I was disappointed that the RCP/BNF Report did not at least warn against the unnecessary introduction of other foods to the breast-fed infant, and that it did not discriminate between exclusively and partially breast-fed children. Complementary feeding of infant formulae is still regarded as safe by many British nurses, when the truth is that it may be extremely harmful (see p. 15).

Another current theory about the causes of colic relates to unnatural interventions (including exposure to drugs) at the time of birth. Colic is simply a disease of medical progress, to be accepted as normal now that over a third of all babies suffer from it. I would agree that there are likely to be such associations, and I agree that we must resist any trend towards increasing intervention in uncomplicated labours. Indeed, as *Breastfeeding Matters* makes clear, I think midwives need to redefine or reassert their role. I applaud these researchers' emphasis on the severity of the stress created by colic and its part in family breakdown. But I disagree that obstetric practices determine whether colic exists. I know many homebirth families with colicky babies (who improved with changes in maternal diet) and many babies who experienced horrific hospital births without becoming colicky, or who had easy births and were colicky and were cured by diet changes. Yet for all that, I would agree that obstetric intervention, drugs, prematurity

30

Food intolerance in infancy

and so on *are* risk factors for colic; indeed, I have argued that we have not yet sorted out how much of the often-adverse outcome for multiples or premature babies is because of their birth condition and how much is caused by different dietary/other consequences that followed from the fact of their being premature or one of multiples. For the truth is that once a baby has experienced difficulty before or during birth, many other things change. The baby is more likely to be separated from its mother, more likely to be given things other than breast-milk (formulae, antibiotics, other drugs), more likely to continue to be stressed by lack of body contact, of non-nutritive sucking, and much more. The mother is more likely to be stressed, with consequent effects on her immune function; more likely to be given drugs of all sorts; more likely to have trouble establishing breast-feeding smoothly and efficiently in harmony with the baby's needs; and so on. All of these things, as well as the stress of the birth, make food intolerance more likely. Hence the response to well-thought-out dietary changes.

My views are not in conflict with these researchers, and I heartily endorse their attempts to call a halt to unnecessarily intrusive obstetric practices. But I must insist on going further, because my approach offers hope of an end to the torment, whereas theirs seems to imply that once the birth has happened like that, you just have to wait till the baby 'grows out of it'. Perhaps in some cases you do. In others, you do not: thousands of families testify to that—not merely Australian families who have written to me or to the Allergy Association, but also New Zealand families involved with the CRY-SOS clinics set up by researchers at Massey University; Scandinavian families; American families being counselled by the Lactation Institute, Encino; English families being helped by London researchers such as Dr Andrew Cant and by the National Childbirth Trust. I could show sceptics a drawer full of such reports. I would be prepared to state confidently that any doctor who has not found that a significant proportion of colicky breast-fed babies are 'cured' by dietary changes either (a) has not tried such change, or (b) has not realized how complex it can sometimes be to find/eliminate the offending foods or chemicals.

A recent French report[16] based on 253 infants, confirmed a higher prevalence of colic in bottle-fed infants, but showed clearly that parental smoking was associated with postprandial (after feeding) colic and other digestive symptoms. Again, this is compatible

31

with the idea of food and chemical intolerance—which Australian mothers so often find is the cause of their babies' colic.

Crying, colic and night waking are only a tiny portion of the range of symptoms which experienced mothers report as disappearing and reappearing with dietary changes—changes in maternal diet, for the breast-feeding mother, or changes in infant diet directly. Symptoms commonly noted in babies[17] are summarized in Table 4.1. Note that this is not intended to be a full list; it omits many serious disorders and many rare ones.

For the parents of the colicky baby, the only real question is how to stop the baby crying. If that is your concern, please try out the ideas on p. 115 and let your local breastfeeding counsellor know whether these ideas helped or not. She may be able to help with practical information, recipes, and contacts. And your experience may assist other parents, and ultimately, even the experts.

DO SUCH MINOR SYMPTOMS MATTER?

These symptoms range from minor oddities to serious problems. In the series of mothers followed up, those who consistently reported the minor symptoms were regarded as neurotic or overprotective. Yet these same mothers found that over months there was often a gradual increase in the severity of symptoms—sometimes dramatically so, as they introduced solids to their child. (The baby who had had tiny patches of dry skin while fully breast-fed suddenly developed eczema, for example.) The question should be asked, would the serious symptoms ever have appeared had the mother identified and avoided the dietary allergen responsible?

Mothers were almost never taken seriously until the child had gross symptoms. In the intervening period of continued exposure, the child had frequently developed multiple intolerances, and even secondary enzyme deficiencies possibly due to the effects on his gut of prolonged exposure to the excitant and resulting immune complexes and chemicals.[16] It is possible that some children might have developed these additional intolerances in any case—but again, leaving them exposed to potential gut damage probably increases the chances. So minor symptoms may matter a great deal.

The child who as a symptom of intolerance has continual frequent loose stools, and who eats well, but gains weight only poorly, may be at greater long-term risk than the child who has severe

Food intolerance in infancy

Table 4.1 Common symptoms in infancy

<table>
<tr><td>

GASTROINTESTINAL TRACT
Frequent possetting or regurgitation
Vomiting, projectile vomiting
Frequent loose stools—mucus
Windiness, excessive flatus
Diarrhoea
Constipation (uncommon in the full breast-fed)
Stomach pains, bloating
Colic
Blood in stools
Poor appetite and weight gain
Feeding difficulties (breast-fed baby often refuses breast after couple of minutes and screams despite obvious hunger. Also rejects bottles.)

RESPIRATORY TRACT
Nasal stuffiness, mucus
Sneezing
Coughing
Nose-rubbing
Unusual breathing
Sniffing, snorting, etc.
Noisy breathing
Hiccoughs
Recurrent croup
Recurrent bronchitis
Frequent ear infections (or any in the fully breast-fed)
Runny nose (clear at first)
Frequent 'colds'
Bad breath

</td><td>

GENITOURINARY TRACT
Cystitis
Vulvovaginitis
Haematuria
Nephrosis

SKIN
Dry patches of skin, cracks
Cradle cap
'Spots'; rashes
Eczema
Hives, welts, swelling (eyes)
Purpura
Scratching or rubbing indicating itchiness
Sweatiness
Redness around mouth, anus, or on cheeks
Easy bruising
Cold hands and feet

CIRCULATION
Changes in pulse rate and regularity, palpitations
Changes in temperature (usually slight fever)
Changes in skin colour, especially around lips
Anaemia, haemolysis
Cold hands and feet

</td></tr>
</table>

diarrhoea. Both states may result in malnutrition. A child can be malnourished because his body simply is not absorbing some essential nutrients in his food. Malabsorption is more readily diagnosed nowadays, but must be considered a possible consequence of neglected intolerance problems.[17] Unfortunately, there has not been any realistic education of parents in developed countries as to the importance of monitoring their child's growth, despite the importance placed on this by the international maternal and child health experts.

Parents should keep in touch with their baby clinic and check that the child's growth curve (on the charts the Sister keeps) remains reasonably steady and in rough proportion to his birth-weight over the months. Isolated parents should keep such records themselves: local health authorities can supply the charts, or good low-cost materials are available from TALC (see p. 197). If these 'percentile' charts show a progressive decline down to the 10th percentile or below, parents should seek specialist help. But don't panic! Children are capable of fantastic rates of catch-up growth once the problem is identified. Only if the problem goes unrecognized for the child's first few years does permanent harm result, and even then the effects are very variable. It is probably a good idea to give these slow-growing children a low-dose, low-allergy vitamin and mineral supplement to ensure against possible deficiencies (see pp. 76–7).

Recurrent bouts of diarrhoea are a problem for very many food-intolerant children. The once-accepted 'treatment'—starvation, flat lemonade, and even drugs—is hazardous for such children. As a consequence a guide to the home management of diarrhoea is included in this edition. Consult your GP before using it, if possible, and buy a packet of oral rehydration salts from the chemist now (Dioralyte and Dextrolyte are two UK brands). (Since Britain has an excellent, if beleaguered, free National Health Service, no parent in the UK should need to 'go it alone' in using these solutions.) Diarrhoea can be very quickly fatal in young children, and you should go to your local hospital if your doctor is unavailable. However, keeping the child well hydrated in the meantime is essential.

CAN IT EVER BE HARMFUL TO BREAST-FEED?

Possibly. A few babies with a particular immune defect *might* develop less allergic disease when bottle-fed from birth. A theory has been advanced that for such babies constant large doses may suppress a faulty immune response, whereas small or intermittent doses may trigger an allergic response.[18] At present this is an academic theory of little relevance to parents because it is imposs-

Food intolerance in infancy

ible to identify these particular children before birth. It would be foolhardy to expose a baby to all the risks of formula feeding so as to minimize a rare cause of allergic disease. After all, it is not yet clear just how much of the immune system is suppressed by constant large doses of foreign protein. What affects one part of the immune response may very well affect another. Hence it is not clear whether resistance to infection is lowered by this aspect of bottle-feeding (as well as others).[19]

Some who discuss this seem unaware of the recent research into human milk and the problems of substitutes. Their own research shows little evidence of any serious investigation of maternal diet in pregnancy and lactation, and history of allergy—or even of neonatal exposure to formula. It may be simply coincidence that almost every mother of a hypersensitive breast-fed baby discovers that she herself was either bottle-fed totally or partially from a very early age, or breast-fed by a smoking mother. But it seems to me like a coincidence that needs testing. Perhaps we are looking at a cumulative effect over generations: after all, each baby has to be born out of a woman's body. And it is a fact that popular advice and medical practice in the management of breast-feeding in preceding generations made the early use of foreign foods almost inevitable.

An undiagnosed food-intolerant mother may sensitize her child *in utero* or via her milk. She herself may benefit, along with baby, from care in diet, etc. To assess the comparative incidence of allergy we need a control group of non-intolerant, healthy, well-nourished mothers who were themselves exclusively breast-fed. I know very few!

One of the few people to look closely at food allergy in the breast-fed infant, Professor J. W. Gerrard, of Canada, suggests that there are two different types of allergy in breast- and bottle-fed children—and that breast-fed babies are more likely to have persistent, sometimes severe, IgE-mediated reactions. (Skin prick tests would be positive.) By contrast, the bottle-fed baby's reaction is probably mediated by IgG or IgM or immune complexes, is less severe, and more usually transient.[20] Checking this theory (based on only 73 children, seen over a period of 25 years) against the experience of the hundreds of families I have dealt with, I find reality more confusing than that. Firstly, it is hard to get exclusively breast- or bottle-fed children—most babies are given some of both in Australia at present. And it is now clear that the effect on gut bacteria is long-lasting, which no-one suspected years ago when comparing breast- and bottle-fed infants. Secondly, the range of reactions varies from trivial to severe in both types, although as we have said, symptom-free periods are quite common and may last years. Are those bottle-fed babies sensitive but currently asymptomatic? What is their long term prognosis? Thirdly, here in Australia skin prick tests have been widely used for both types of babies, and are more often negative than positive in both, even when the children are clearly milk-intolerant. Fourthly, the severity of the mother's childhood problems, shorter birth intervals and increasing parity all seem to be associated with increasing severity of the baby's reactions whether breast- or bottle-fed. So maternal factors may decide which children, however fed, show symptoms that are IgE mediated.

Now that is purely impressionistic: I cannot quantify and tabulate that data without resources I simply do not have. But if my impressions are accurate, it may be because I have been dealing with whole families whose initially perceived problem was a colicky baby, not 'allergy'. Most were certainly not sick enough for their doctor to send them to a hospital-based research specialist such as Professor Gerrard. It seems probable to me that the community end of the food-intolerance spectrum is a lot more diverse and confusing than the specialist can hope to see. Professor Gerrard saw only 27 such babies over a two-year period, despite his well known interest in the subject. We could however both be right because we are looking at different ends of the elephant, like the blind men in the fable.

Professor Gerrard sees the breast-fed baby's ability to respond to trace amounts of antigen as possibly advantageous in evolutionary terms. 'IgE is known to play an important role . . . in the primary immune response, at least to rival antigens. To be effective in this role IgE must be produced in the very early stages of an infection, when antigenic exposure is minimal. Those who respond best to minimal, low-dose stimulation can be expected to mount the most rapid, and presumably effective, immune response.'[21] In other words, if it happens in breast-fed babies, there's quite possibly a good reason for it to happen!

However, there seem to me to be real problems in deciding what is a small dose and what is not. Possibly breast-feeding mothers on

Food intolerance in infancy

identical diets excrete quite different amounts and types of antigen or other chemical mediators of allergic responses. Is there perhaps a threshold level of antigen(s) in breast milk, which excites a response—qualities below that threshold can be deemed 'small', and those above, large enough to cause trouble? This would explain why some mothers who tried the diet advice for subsequent pregnancies (given in section two) found that their new babies did not respond as older siblings had to accidental diet infringements. Many such mothers were able to have modest amounts of milk, for example, without obvious problems in the baby. There must be some mechanism which explains why every breast-fed baby does not produce IgE reactions to every food in the mother's diet! So the question of dose-related response seems to me much more complicated than anyone has yet ventured to raise. The variables may include: degree of permeability of maternal and infant gut; degree of inherited immune defect; relative rates of excretion of antigen in milk; quantities ingested by mother and child (of breast milk at any one feed); relative amounts of other substances in breast milk which might enhance, modulate, or block certain responses, and so on. I simply do not think we can talk of breast-feeding as though there were no variables in that very individual process. Nor indeed is 'bottle-feeding' a uniform process. Formulae vary wildly in their protein content and allergenicity, osmolality, and much more. Perhaps studies discussing bottle-feeding should specify what formula, and append its current composition? (Preferably its composition as measured by an independent laboratory, too.)

Further support for the idea that it is not breast-feeding *per se*, but breast-feeding by an already affected baby might be suggested by the results of one report[22] on 72 six-year-olds allergic to cows' milk. 60 per cent had a family history of allergy and were bottle-fed; 26 per cent had a family history of allergy and were breast-fed; 14 per cent had no family history. ALL of that 14 per cent were bottle-fed. Breast-feeding was almost certainly not exclusive from birth, yet no breast-fed child became cows' milk allergic unless allergy was already in the family. This would fit neatly with the idea that it may be the second and succeeding generations who are most adversely affected by unphysiological infant feeding practices. To find breast-fed babies who suffer from cows' milk allergy/intolerance when there is no history of family allergy, and no

37

Food for thought

history of maternal dietary aberrations or early infant exposure in either generation, would be interesting. I am sure such families exist, because there are so many pathways to intolerance; but I suspect that they may be rare.

Of course if must also be remembered that allergy is not the only concern in decisions about whether to breast-feed. Optimal brain growth, proper development, long-term health are also important—here human milk wins easily.[23] But it could happen that a mother might need to find other sources of human milk, for example, if she had severe intolerance problems, smoked heavily, and could not solve those problems. And I say other sources of *human* milk intentionally, however impracticable that may seem at present, and despite the unexplored potential hazards[24] involved in using milk from other mothers. My first choice in such a devastating situation would be to explore the possibility of wet-nursing. As Soothill says, 'Passive transfer of human milk is the most physiological, and the longest standing alternative to breastfeeding by the mother. . . .'[25] It has always been common in human society; it is still going on, although rarely mentioned, in Australia,[26] and no doubt in England too, though to a lesser extent I suspect. But UK research into human milk banking and milk modification is far ahead of us in Australia—and using banked, modified human milk would be my second choice if finding a suitable wet-nurse proved impossible.

However, there is a tiny minority of babies born with congenital abnormalities or with such a degree of sensitivity to contaminants or components of human milk that breast-feeding is completely ruled out, and a highly specialized and costly formula must be used. In two cases I have known—both children of smokers, which may be pure chance or may not—weaning on to such formulae meant rapid improvement. This cannot be relied upon—in other cases babies became rapidly worse. Also those two children were 8 months or older—perhaps that helped them. If your baby is weaned on to such formulae, and thrives, rejoice and thank modern science with a clear conscience—your main responsibility is to see that the child eats and grows well, and if you cannot supply his needs yourself, that is nothing to feel guilty about. The reasons *why* you can't are certainly complex and equally certainly *not* your entire responsibility. The point of infant feeding, as Gunther said, is to feed the infant, not to satisfy maternal urges or needs (though it may do that too).

Food intolerance in infancy

All the same, weaning may not solve your problems, especially if weaning is suggested by someone who has not really investigated you and the baby in any careful detail. Therefore remember to hedge your bets. Prior to, or after, weaning you can organize a supply of frozen milk; you can continue to express in case you decide to relactate (see p. 39). But remember that even if you don't express you can still relactate simply by letting baby suckle the breast, although it is more difficult. Advice on relactation can be had from the National Childbirth Trust (NCT) or from La Leche League International (LLLI) (see p. 198). Various devices exist which can help. But your principal necessity when considering relactation is a 'doula', someone supportive and encouraging. This may be your husband, your mother, or a counsellor from one of the breast-feeding mothers support groups.

WHAT IS WRONG WITH INFANT FORMULA?

It is time that some of the known facts about formula feeding were made public—because many parents are blissfully ignorant of the hazards, and see the choice as one of no great moment. It is undeniable that many children grow and thrive normally—as the culture defines normally—when fed artificial formulae. (It is also undeniable that we don't know how those children might have been different had they been fed breast milk—would they have been taller or shorter, spoken more clearly, been more intelligent, less obese, lived longer, had less disease or fewer food-intolerant babies? etc.—these are imponderables, although some interesting research goes on.) Again, I don't want to alarm parents who from choice, mismanagement, or necessity bottle-fed their children—as I have said before, the responsibility is not yours, and most children, however fed, are acceptably healthy and bright. But for *some* children it matters a great deal. And since it's impossible to know before birth whether your child is going to be one of those, the hazards need to be stated—because almost no-one else will tell you this, for fear of upsetting you.

FACT 1. **Formula feeding provides no immunological protection against disease for your baby**; in fact it encourages the growth of harmful bowel bacteria. It is said that some companies are currently thinking of adding gamma-globulin to formula in order to

39

advertise that they now provide such protection. This will probably turn out to be impracticable or even unwise (and who are to be the guinea-pigs?). In any case gamma-globulin will not do a fraction of what your milk does (for more detail see Lawrence, *Breastfeeding, A guide for the medical profession*, Chapter 5). Did you know that your body can make specific antibodies for every bacteria or virus that threatens your baby; that you supply interferon among the many other active ingredients of your milk? Drug companies cannot compete here—their products are not so highly specific, and therefore almost always have side effects.

FACT 2. **Formula feeding is based upon our limited knowledge of the components of human milk,** with extra added for safety. It represents a sort of average plus, and after the first few days simply increases in volume as baby grows. (The relative amounts of ingredients do not change at all.) The composition of breast milk changes during a feed, over a day, and over months—so much so that milk from the mother of a 6-month-old baby will not promote optimal (i.e. best possible) growth of a 6-week-old baby. The milk of a mother delivered prematurely, and the mother weaning her baby, have very different quantities of certain constituents. Human milk changes as baby grows. Formula cannot, unless the manufacturers start making many different formulae labelled '1st week of life', '2 weeks to one month', etc. And in any case, we don't yet know all that is in human milk—unlike cows' milk, it has not yet been exhaustively studied, being of no commercial interest. What we know about milk always reflects the current limitations of the technology (and the researchers) investigating it. Yet each new brand has been advertised as virtually the same as mother's milk—even ones that would be illegal under current draft standards.[27] All such formulae were considered safe—once.

FACT 3. **Formula feeding is inexact**. You *never* know what baby is getting, even though you can see how many ounces of white fluid goes in. If the scoop is pressed too hard, or not firmly enough, the resultant changes in composition can be significant. When breastfeeding you don't have to worry—it is all done for you. The idea that 'you know how much a bottlefed baby is getting' is laughable—how much of what?

Food intolerance in infancy

FACT 4. **Formula feeding is for a mythical average baby.** Is *your* baby growing too big because he is overfed, or not big enough because he is underfed? Is he thirsty and needs more water or hungry and needs more food? In breast-feeding these problems sort themselves out—in hot weather, for example, your milk becomes more dilute if baby suckles more frequently. If he is only thirsty but feeds more often it won't matter because the low solute load of breast milk won't harm his immature kidneys. Extra formula puts great strain on his body.

FACT 5. **Formula feeding is subject to human error**, both in the formulation and the preparation of what is put into the can. Because it is big business, when troubles show up they are not always publicized or rectified. A *partial* list of some very recent tragic mistakes follows:—a more complete account can be found in Dr Neil Campbell's excellent article.[28]

(a) Essential fatty acid deficiency in some formulae caused skin, eye, and gut disorders, and failure to thrive.

(b) Too much iron in some formulae caused gastrointestinal bleeding, anaemia, and immunological disorders.

(c) Lead contaminates all canned formulae when the solder used in the cans is lead. Lead damages the brain, and is a cumulative poison.

(d) In the late 1970s an Australian manufacturer knowingly sold overseas infant formula contaminated with salmonella bacteria; it had caused widespread illness in Australia before being identified.

(e) The tough, indigestible curds formed from the protein in some formulae caused bowel obstruction requiring surgery in some babies. (It is these tough curds which enable some bottle-fed babies to 'last' 4 hours between feeds.) A formula newly marketed in 1978, designed for premature babies, was one that had this effect.

(f) In 1978 Enfamil with iron (made in the USA) was recalled because it was green, curdled, sour, and contained dangerous bacteria. (At least in this case mothers could see something peculiar.)

(g) In 1980 Soy-a-lac and 1-soy-a-lac were recalled because they contained too much vitamin D, which can be toxic, causing convulsions and kidney damage.

Food for thought

(h) In 1979, Neo-mull-soy and Cho-free (Syntex) were found to lack chloride. The result was metabolic alkalosis—failure to thrive, constipation, diarrhoea and vomiting, dehydration, lethargy, developmental delays, mild retardation, convulsions, cerebral palsy, kidney defects.[29] Consumer groups in the USA have not been able to discover whether the defective formula was exported after the ban. (Why not?)

(i) In the last few years, biotin has been added to most infant formulae, after it was discovered that animals dying from what seemed like sudden infant death syndrome, or cot death, were very deficient in biotin.

(j) The latest recall of defective infant formula took place in the USA only in 1985. Now the US Food and Drug Administration is required by law to routinely test all infant formulae to see that what is on the label is indeed contained in the tin.

In the UK, a report in 1980 laid down some guidelines for manufacturers, which doubtless the reputable concerns are following. But all such guidelines must represent a compromise between what is commercially possible and relatively inexpensive, and what is currently known about human milk. Using cows' milk, coconut oil, and the rest it is simply not possible to construct an exact duplicate of human milk.[30] (Even if it were, which human milk would be duplicated: that at 6 days, 6 weeks, 6 months, or which?) There is a point beyond which formula becomes too expensive, and human milk banking and wet-nursing the only commercial option.[31] But consider the impact on primary industry if cows' milk is to be seen as unsuitable for young babies! Naturally it was the Department of Primary Industry which consulted with the manufacturers to work out a voluntary code to put 'the aims and principles' (but not the specifics??) of the WHO Code into effect in Australia. Despite repeated requests, consumer representation was not allowed. Similarly, the UK Code, drawn up by the Food Manufacturers' Federation, is voluntary and significantly weaker than the WHO Code. Its weakness was very obvious as I visited hospitals in the UK: the constant presence of 'gifts' from infant-formula companies added up to a professional endorsement of formula in the eyes of new mothers. (Contact the NCT for details of their concern over the FMF Code.)

Food intolerance in infancy

Until EEC legislation is adopted, even such codes as exist have no teeth. Are health food shops selling inadequate goats' milk powders for infant use? These imports turn up in Australia—who is monitoring the situation in the UK? How rapidly are recalls of formula in the USA communicated to export markets such as the UK? And why is it that there are so few publicized recalls of Australian and UK products? Is this because manufacturing processes are intrinsically safer outside the USA, or is it that the US Food and Drug Administration exercises a more detailed control and surveillance of manufactured goods? Do *we* rarely have recalls because the mechanism for checking formulae do not exist?

Of course, even when a formula is defective, the results will not be disastrous for every child. Since humans are amazingly adaptable, most babies are able to adjust to less than optimal diets, and grow adequately. We simply cannot provide an absolutely optimal diet and environment for all children—on a world scale, we are not even providing an adequate one for most children. So minor defects in formulae may be seen as trivial from that perspective. However, the consequences are not always trivial—hence the need to avoid the risk wherever humanly possible. If it is *not* humanly possible to avoid the risk of formulae, then one must be philosophical—and grateful that the risks in 1984 are probably less than they have ever been. Even so, let us not kid ourselves that adequate growth is optimal growth, despite the images created by clever advertising. (Were the babies used to advertise a formula fed exclusively on that formula from birth? I doubt it.) In using formula, we are accepting second best—inevitable sometimes, but never a matter for rejoicing or pride.

The truth about formula feeding is that it represents an uncontrolled *in vivo* experiment on very vulnerable humans;[32] that accident and ignorance in its preparation have caused a great deal of avoidable sickness and death in the last hundred years; and that we are only beginning now to ask questions about the long-term impact of such an experiment on the pattern of chronic disease in our society. It is currently thought to be a trifle extreme, even fanatical, to question such a 'normal' method of infant feeding. The pity is, that no-one thought to question its introduction before it became 'normal'. Our faith in 'scientific' formulations has been exceeded only by our unwillingness to ask hard questions about

43

the sorts of social changes that made bottle-feeding seem necessary or attractive to our parents' generation.

To put matters into another perspective—despite the strong commercial pressures towards early weaning in intensive pig farming, it has proved to be uneconomic to wean piglets before 3 weeks (that is, around one-third of the normal lactation cycle). Too many piglets fail to thrive, or die. Many still do, but these are compensated for by the extra litter that mother pig can produce once weaned and impregnated again. No doubt with intravenous feeding, drug therapy, and so on, many of the more vulnerable piglets could be saved—but the cost is excessive.

Could it be that it is only the massive expansion of our hospital system over the last century which has prevented us from seeing the real impact in *developed* countries of formula feeding for infants? Would infantile gastroenteritis, for example, come to be seen as an avoidable disease, a rarity, rather than as a major cause of infant admissions to hospital, once breast-feeding is again universal? This is a realistic goal, once the medical profession is resolute in promoting it, and consumers in demanding it. The experience of Dr Relucio-Clavano, at Baguio General Hospital proves this to any interested person. Not one baby, however ill or premature, receives anything but human milk and the comparative morbidity (sickness) and mortality figures for the period before and after the total ban on formula are staggeringly different.[33]

Of course there were, and will be, a small percentage of mothers who could not breast-feed successfully—but because all the others were feeding, there was no problem in obtaining human milk for their babies. Infancy is a time of rapid brain growth—surely only the breast will do!

And surely too, feminists will soon come to see how much of a feminist issue infant feeding really is. The image of the breast-feeding mother may have been associated in the past with domestic confinement; it could just as easily nowadays be seen as the only truly liberated style of feeding. It is perfectly possible to breast-feed exclusively for at least 5 months (by means of careful organization) while being actively employed or job-sharing.[34] Where it is not possible, the lack of decent facilities, or sufficient lactation leave (why not paid, as it is in some countries?) should be matters for union action.[35] Feminists need not compromise their principles to actively promote breast-feeding—indeed one could argue that to allow woman's own original product to be supplanted by the products of commercial enterprises is to betray feminist principle. As Elisabet Helsing pointed out at the April 1984 breast-feeding seminar organized by the International College of Midwives, Norwegian feminists have always supported breast-feeding.[36] Ann Oakley has written a marvellous article on this subject.[37]

Although this is a lengthy piece, it is only a fraction of what might be said about the differences between breast and substitutes. All the rest will be in the next book I am writing, *Breastfeeding Matters*.

WHAT FOODS ARE MOST LIKELY TO CAUSE TROUBLE?

In our culture, first and foremost, milk. Allergens are culturally determined—fish and soya are probably far more of a problem in Japan than the UK, for example. Milk is undoubtedly a marvellous food for those who are tolerant of it. But milk products are everywhere in English foods—in bread, margarine, many processed foods, even hamburgers—and the market for milk by-products is ever increasing. This may make economic sense; for many people it is nutritional disaster. And above all, the untested, indiscriminate use of milk in the first few months of infant lives is the problem: not milk itself. Should someone decide that peanut butter was an immensely valuable food and create a fad for feeding that to babies, we could expect a generation of peanut-intolerant babies! In fact, any food or other chemical combination given to the newborn baby can both sensitize and cause the same problems as cows' milk. Note the list of common allergens below,[38] and compare it with foods given to babies directly or via the breast-feeding mother's milk.

Orange juice deserves a special mention: allergists urge that it not be given to children under 12 or 18 months, yet in some places it is urged upon even breast-fed babies under 6 months, in the mistaken notion that breast milk does not contain enough vitamin C.[39] Paediatric syrups of all kinds are loaded with artificial colourings, flavourings, and preservatives—all clearly implicated in hyperactivity problems in many older children; yet given blithely

Food for thought

Table 4.2 Common allergens in Western diet

Common allergens in Western diet	Less common but not rare allergens
Cows' milk	Legumes, nuts, potato, tomato
Dairy products—cheese	(especially sauce)
Eggs	Corn products
Fish	Tinned food (if left in tin after
	opening)
Wheat—especially bleached white	
flour	Frozen food (frequently has
	additives)
Cane sugar	Root vegetables
Artificial colouring	Spices
Preservatives	Yeast
Soya	Chocolate, cocoa, coffee, tea
[Yeast]	Wine (especially red) and
[Citrus fruits]	alcoholic drinks

Reproduced from von Witt, V.–Chronic illness and hidden food allergies. *Modern Medicine*, July 1978, 8–14.

as a 'help' for the weary mother of the colicky child. The relationship between original cows' milk intolerance and later Feingold-type hypersensitivities should really be investigated now that the neurobiologists and neurochemists have begun serious and very promising research into the biological activity of food dyes and additives.[40] Although this is another area of not-yet-proven facts, it is interesting to read journals like *Pediatrics* and notice that Mead Johnson manufactures additive-free and alcohol-free drugs for asthmatics in the US.[41]

Then there's the use of cereals for babies. This has been linked with the rise of coeliac disease, an intolerance to the gluten in cereal. After concern was expressed in 1974–5 in the UK about current infant feeding practices the Government conducted a national campaign to improve the quality of nutritional advice and help with breast-feeding given to mothers. The results?—a progressive increase in breast-feeding, improvement in artificial feeding practices and later introduction of solids—and a steady decline ever since of gluten intolerance.[42] If, as this suggests, coeliac disease is linked with childhood diet, the problem is at least partly preventable—what mother would give cereal to her tiny baby if

46

Food intolerance in infancy

she had been told of the possible consequences? Once again, the notion that one must not make any mother feel guilty, (see p. 81) becomes justification for inaction and so greater harm. (I said justification—should I have said excuse?)

WOULD SOY MILK OR GOATS' MILK BE BETTER FOR CHILDREN?

That may depend on a number of factors. If this means 'from birth', the answer is no. Babies given soy milks from birth have roughly comparable rates of allergic disease.[43] Cows'-milk-intolerant babies switched abruptly to other milks are also not very likely to benefit—if the cow's milk has damaged a child's gut, it is quite likely that he will also be sensitive to soy used in the same massive quantities.

None the less, it is clear that some babies are a lot better on soy or goats' milk. This may be because soya bean milk contains essential fatty acids in which the child is deficient (see p. 80).[44] It may also be because they are that much older when the change is made, and can cope with the new diet, perhaps partly because in pregnancy goat and soy protein were not over-indulged in. It may also be because being older, the child is on a more varied diet which reduces the total quantity of any one food, or ingredients of which interact and help with digestion of soy or goats' milk. Many children refuse to have large quantities of soy or goats' milk, and parents accept that more easily because the taste is worse, and the product more expensive, than cows' milk. It may also be though, that the child's intolerance of the new food is unrecognized because the symptoms change, and are not as awful as the previous ones. To swap constant nightwaking for a runny nose may seem a small price to pay!

So far I have met many parents who have tried alternatives, but very few who are really sure that the child is completely unaffected by the substitute. In some cases intolerance emerges only slowly. The nutritional benefit of the substitute may outweigh its disadvantage too—again a personal decision.

All the same, it is clear that modified goats' milk, despite its similarity to cows' milk, has enabled many babies to survive over generations. Research may yet discover that it is of some value in this field—and perhaps sheep's milk too. But there are definite

Food for thought

hazards in using these substitutes. High standards of hygiene are critical, especially if you buy them raw, or unpasteurized. Few people realize that extremely nasty diseases such as brucellosis and toxoplasmosis can be contracted from untreated animal milks. The sickness and death caused by improper handling and storage of milk in the days before pasteurization and herd control is almost beyond belief. So make sure that your milk comes from herds which have been vaccinated, and that there is some quality control over the pasteurization process. If in any doubt, consult your health visitor, clinic sister, or doctor, and follow their directions. Never give babies raw animal milks: yes, there is a loss of nutrients in boiling milk, but the loss of micro-organisms makes up for it! And boiling reduces its ability to sensitize as well.[45] However, once heated, milk will spoil faster, as the natural systems that retard bacterial growth have been destroyed, so you must be scrupulously careful to throw away any left-over milk in the bottle, and to refrigerate the rest.

Animal milks are often deficient in something—goats' milk in folic acid, for example. This needs to be added to your diet in some form if goats' milk is a major constituent. For this and other reasons, *home made formulae are definitely out for young babies*. As the Department of Health and Social Security stated, 'goats' milk preparations should be given to infants only under medical supervision.' They are not suitable for children under 6 months of age, any more than cows' milk is.

Soyabean milks also have their problems. As with other milks, you cannot make at home an adequate diet for the young infant, without access to the guide in Helsing and King (see p. 122). You need to know about fatty acids, limiting amino acids, and much more. . . . But the soy formulae too are an experiment, and a more recent experiment at that, so opinion in the medical profession is very divided as to whether they are more or less suitable than cows' milk formulae. The RCP/BNF Joint Report was quite clear: 'There is no justification for recommending soy milks instead of cows' milk formulae. . . . There may even be a contraindication to soy-based formula feeding, in that it results in poor antibody responses to immunization.'[46] Never use soy flours without proper cooking, too, as they contain natural substances which damage the gut lining and inhibit the enzymes which digest nutrients—as a result, the protein is not available to the child. (A fact

48

Food intolerance in infancy

pointed out by the failure of some babies to thrive on early soy formulae.)

As I travel about the country I hear of all sorts of other substitutes in use, particularly nut milks. None of these is suitable for very young babies, or as the major part of the diet of an older child, without scrupulous nutiritional oversight. What little we do know about infant feeding points out the need for very complicated formulation of breast milk substitutes. If cows' milk is unsuitable as a sole food for anything but calves, so are all these other milks unsuitable for human infants. They may have their uses, but if a baby is not being breast-fed he needs a good 'scientific' formula.

Other substitutes are currently being marketed for the whole family. One, Meadowfresh, claims to be lower in allergens, and a boon to the milk-sensitive, despite being formulated from milk whey (and many other ingredients). So far I have heard only from the distributors. It would seem likely that some families might be helped by it. It would also seem likely that others would not, as the whey proteins are among the most potent milk allergens. I will be interested to hear from parents who are not distributors: can your children tolerate it without symptoms? how long have you used if for? how much is used each day? and so on.

5

Inhalant problems

So far I have not yet encountered a family that has food but not inhalant problems, or vice versa. (Quite a few families had no hayfever last spring when the only change they had made was to eliminate a few foods.) Concentrating on food intolerances is not meant to imply that these are more important than inhalant or chemical problems. However, no one denies that inhalants cause problems; the idea that food does is still relatively unpopular. Food intolerance is seriously under-diagnosed, although many parents consider it the easiest part of their family total body load to manipulate and control. Reducing any part of the total body load is likely to help prevent or reduce symptoms, so if environmental modification is possible and considered easier than diet, it is as good a place as any to begin.

For inhalational excitants the remedies are the same as those for dietary ones—avoidance where possible, and desensitization techniques. Some drugs are also helpful in relieving attacks, but are too often used instead of basic preventative self-help measures. This could leave the person with an extremely high total body load very vulnerable to severe attacks, and a few deaths result every year from such attacks.

The major causes of inhalant-linked disease are:

Animal fur, feathers, hair, dander, etc.—pets, bedding, stuffing of toys, house dust (containing tiny mites, one of the most potent common allergens. Increasing evidence suggests that even very young babies may be reacting to dust-mite. Parents who use lambskins ought to follow care instructions about the frequency of shaking and washing, or cover the lambskin with a cotton sheet. Lambskins are good for babies, but dust-mites are not.)
Plant products—includes grasses and pollens—worse at different seasons and in different areas. Foods such as flours, rolled cereals,

50

Inhalant problems

etc. may cause similar problems when dust is inhaled. Tobacco. Moulds.

Chemicals of all descriptions. Common household chemicals should be used as sparingly as possible or not at all, and kept outside the house. Slow release pesticides are taboo—they accumulate in body fat and may then pass into breast milk; or to be released in toxic quantities if the person loses weight suddenly. Soaps, detergents, and so on should be as simple as possible. Perfumes and cosmetics often cause problems. Cigarettes always do (see p. 52). Industrial pollution and car exhausts will usually affect such children badly. Other possibilities—chlorine in swimming pools (especially enclosed ones), gas and oil heating, plastics (furniture, toys), felt marker pens, fresh newsprint or other duplicated paper (sometimes important for schoolchildren), synthetic bedding and pillows (often implicated in night-time headaches and nosebleeds), and so on. The list is virtually endless. For detailed advice in this area, see Natalie Golo's book, *Coping with your allergies*, or Doris Rapp's *Allergies and your family*, pp. 188–94.

There is substantial intertwining of these three categories. Plant extracts are often used in chemicals, as are animal products. All may be used in foods in some cases. A person may have both an inhalational and a dietary allergy to related products. Simple precautions include a reasonably dust-free house, pets only outside if at all, as few chemicals as possible, dust- and allergen-free bedrooms. However, to track down these environmental excitants is far more complex than to manipulate diet, and can require specialist help. For further reading see the bibliography (p. 213). Asthma self-help groups often produce helpful free literature, especially on inhalants, the most obvious cause of asthma. The role of diet and chemicals in producing asthma has been less-well recognized until quite recently.[1]

Chemicals deserve a special mention. Almost everyone working with intolerant patients has come to see chemical pollution—of our food, our water, our homes and workplaces, our air—as being a major cause of food intolerance. People who have been exposed in industrial accidents, agriculture, factory, or war, commonly develop food intolerances which may be severe enough to produce gross behavioural changes. (Chemical victims frequently have brain and central nervous system effects.) Whether this is due to some derangement of their immune system, or simply the direct

51

toxicity of the chemical, is not yet clear. In the USA, this problem is far worse, despite the more stringent controls being imposed as its significance is recognized.

It can be unnerving to realize that you have problems on all these fronts, if indeed you do. Try to remember two things. Firstly, this is to be expected and is undoubtedly normal to some degree for everyone, because each person lives in a particular environment with which he interacts. You are unusual only in knowing more about some of those interactions. Secondly, you only have to modify some exposures, not all, to be able to cope better. Therefore you can choose to modify those which are easiest for you. One person may choose the allergy-free bedroom, avoidance of preservatives and monosodium glutamate, and reduction in excessive milk intake. Another may prefer to adopt regular exercise and total milk exclusion. What you do depends on your lifestyle and sensitivities. It will take time to work it out, but once key factors are identified life is better, not worse, for the change.

WHAT IS WRONG WITH SMOKING?

If you are interested to know about this in detail, write to Johns Hopkins University for their free Population Report, *Tobacco —Hazards to health and human reproduction*.[2] Although published in 1979, any news since then has only confirmed the risks they so depressingly outlined. In short, the news is bad. Most people now accept their statement that smoking in pregnancy is associated with lower birth weights, higher rates of spontaneous abortion, especially during later pregnancy, more frequent complications of pregnancy and labour, and higher rates of early infant death. Additionally, there is evidence of increased congenital abnormalities. Infants of smoking parents are more likely to be hospitalized, more likely to suffer bronchitis or pneumonia, and possibly more likely to die of 'cot death'—or Sudden Infant Death Syndrome (SIDS)—though the latter is such an emotive topic that very few researchers will say so publicly, for fear of creating guilt feelings in those smoking parents whose child may have died. (Similarly bottle-feeding is probably a risk factor for SIDS—this is well discussed by Cunningham.[3] And many parents commented on 'peculiar breathing' and snuffles in intolerant breast-fed babies exposed intermittently to either cows' milk or some other allergen—or cigarette smoke.)

Cigarettes and babies don't mix. The breast-feeding smoker provides her baby with a potent cocktail of over four thousand chemical compounds to breathe in or drink. Over 30 of these, including a radioactive element, polonium 210, are known or suspected health hazards. Add to that the fact that tobacco crops are heavily sprayed with pesticides, including DDT, and residues are present in every cigarette, to be absorbed by mother and baby alike. If the smoking mother loses weight while breast-feeding, she also liberates her body stores of fat-soluble toxic compounds. (It is theoretically possible to poison oneself by such sudden liberation of accumulated toxins, and some maintain that it has indeed happened.[4] Drastic weight losses during lactation are obviously not a good idea, even, if like most of us, you pine to be your old shape once again.)

There have been those who have argued that because breast-feeding allows for the excretion of such harmful substances, it could be safer to bottle-feed. Once again, this is a question of relative risks. You do have some control over your own pesticide and drug intake. However, you have none over the intake of the cows whose milk is processed for formula. Simple measures such as thorough washing and/or peeling of fruit, reducing or eliminating household and agricultural pesticides, avoiding recently sprayed areas, reducing consumption of animals fats—and large fishes such as shark—and NO SMOKING, can substantially reduce your everyday burden ot toxic chemicals. If you have been working in high-risk occupations, and are concerned that the levels in your body could be harmful, it might be worth getting tests done to see just what those levels are. Even so, there is no automatic damage to the child—the follow-up of the Michigan families accidentally poisoned via the food chain after stock feed was contaminated, has so far revealed no adverse effects in breast-fed babies. The consensus is that despite high body levels, breast-feeding is still the safest course to follow.[5]

Smoking too may reduce milk production—though this is so variable among women that only those like me with chronic low supply problems (or those particularly sensitive to tobacco, perhaps) might notice the problem. It does alter some constituents of milk, but no-one is sure whether the changes are significant.[6] It

53

Food for thought

probably increases your need for vitamins, especially vitamins B and C.

If you can't quit—at least consider every cigarette and decide whether it is worth it to you. And don't smoke just before or during feeds. If you can't give it up altogether, accept that for now, but keep working on it. There seemed to be a correlation between those cases severe enough to need hospitalization, and parental smoking. This may be coincidence. But some mothers were very angry to realize that this might be a contributory factor—they had asked their doctors whether smoking was OK and got the standard—'don't feel guilty about it—you may need it—no scientific proof that ten a day does any harm—' or whatever. All are non-smokers now. They were motivated to try harder by the evidence.

It should be emphasized that it is also harmful for fathers to smoke, even though they are not supplying milk to the baby. Any father who wants his child to be as healthy, as tall and intelligent as possible must try to keep cigarette smoke outside the child's environment. If at all possible, try to give it up altogether, and you increase your own prospects for a longer, healthier life—and decrease the chance that your children will take up smoking as teenagers.[7] (Or earlier—as intelligent adults move away from smoking, the child and teenage market is increasing, which manufacturers asset is none of their doing. . . . Pity the children of those exploited youngers!)

Naturally, if mother and father are not smoking, they will also try to persuade other relatives and friends not to poison the child's environment. Once again, you explain that the basis for your request is medical; that you are not judging the person who smokes but merely asking that he do so in such a way that he harms only himself. It is very hard at first but when you stay awake all night with a croupy, wheezy child who is suffering because you did not feel you could say anything to the smokers, you toughen up fairly fast! Most people are reasonable about this—and if they are not, then you avoid them. After all, a case is now on record of a child dying of asthma triggered by an adult who lit a cigarette when sitting beside the child.

Don't dismiss all this as scare-mongering because you know Doctor X who smokes, so it can't be that bad. . . . People in high-pressure professions are more likely to turn to stimulants and relaxants of all kinds—and just as likely as anyone else to become addicted to their poisons. The addict, be he doctor or drop-out, faces formidable withdrawal problems. Overall, there has been a *massive* decline in the number of doctors who smoke. Most of the major medical organizations are coming out very strongly against the hypocrisy of governments which subsidize tobacco growing.[8] accept huge revenues from cigarette sales, and then put silly little warnings on the packet—while paying huge costs for medical problems directly caused by smoking. So if your doctor smokes, he is one of the few left who do. Nurses, unfortunately, still have a very high incidence of smokers in their ranks, which is regarded as a major health problem by medical authorities. It also helps explain why so many hospitals still allow, or turn a blind eye to, smokers in the wards. Such nurses sometimes refuse to believe patients who say that cigarette smoke makes them sick, and even punish the victim for complaining!

6

Medical treatments

The most basic diagnostic tool of the practising allergist is a very detailed history-taking session, in which he traces the person's health from birth. The symptoms he discovers become the starting-point of further testing. Although testing has improved over the last decade or so, and become far more sophisticated, there still is no 100 per cent certain, accurate diagnostic test for the wide battery of substances humans can be intolerant of. Indeed, the review of all current methods of testing in the RCP/BNF Joint Report makes this crystal clear. By far the most useful is the controlled challenge, where the person is given food after a period of avoidance, and observed for reactions. However, even this is NOT infallible. If you stop and think for a moment about the endless permutations and combinations of total body load and current tolerance level, you will know why. The person may not be given a sufficient amount, or for a sufficiently long period; the so-called placebo may turn out to be just as allergenic; other variables may have altered, for example, in the largely dust-free hospital environment, a child may cope with milk far better than at home, etc. *ad infinitum* (see pp. 16–17).

Hence the use of different types of test—skin, RAST, cytotoxic, sublingual, etc.—which again usually only strengthen the likelihood that the problems obvious from the history are the major ones. (The tests often pick up some unexpected suspects too, some of which are later confirmed by challenge, and others of which are not).[1] New tests are often hailed as significant advances. The LIF test is one, breath hydrogen another. Each of these tests has its advocates and its critics, and reputable doctors simply do not agree about the worth of any of them. Which your child may be exposed to will depend on the current ideas of the doctors he is referred to. Because of this controversy, not all treatments will be available on

56

Medical treatments

the NHS. This is understandable given the enormous potential for abuse of such tests by those cashing in on the latest fad. Most Western countries have been through some very costly scandals, some involving multiple pathology tests. While I am in sympathy with those who seek to protect the taxpayer and the patient from charlatans, I am not always sure that patients are being listened to. There is a strong danger of creating, or reinforcing, a two-tiered health system, where health insurance determines access to all sorts of testing denied to others. There is also a danger that tests which *do* work for *some* will be denounced as useless because they do not *always* work for *everybody*. If doctors and patients were enabled to communicate better, that is, more honestly, more frequently, and more respectfully, doctors might learn that some tests for which there is as yet no scientific basis were actually helpful clinically; that others which were more respectable scientifically proved to be useless in the long run—or vice versa! I am strongly of the opinion that doctors should be actively seeking patient feedback; involving laymen in conferences, and so on. Patients too would have more chance of understanding the 'orthodox' views of the time, and would be more likely to avoid the rogues and charlatans if they felt that they had been taken seriously by the orthodox. The danger of increasing litigation by parents would also be reduced.

I have not written in any detail about these tests because the debate is so constant and unresolved. One doctor has written that 'at present, identification of allergens in a patient requires a mixture of experience and clairvoyance'! If a doctor is ordering a test for your child, find out what it is, what it involves, what it costs, what his estimate of its usefulness is, whether he considers it essential or merely interesting. Then balance that against the effects on the child and the risks of the procedure. Remember that the child is yours, and that responsibility for decision-making cannot be handed over to anyone else, however authoritative, except in extreme emergencies. If these tests established your child's problem definitively, it would be easier to justify them—but as I have said earlier, none is infallible.

If the tests are part of a research project, other questions should be raised. Most parents are willing to do anything to help doctors who are searching for answers to these problems, and I certainly do not want to discourage research. However, reading the medical

Food for thought

journals has cured me of any inclination to agree automatically to such requests.[2] Children have been subjected to considerable discomfort and even risk in research projects that were not very well designed in the first place, even if they were 'double-blind'. As a result their experience was not worthwhile, and their parents are now rather disillusioned. So if you are asked to take part in a research project, find out exactly what it is designed to test and how this will be done in detail. This is your right. Most research is supposed to be based on 'informed consent', so you should be well informed before you consent. Then think about it in relation to your child at this point in time. If there seem to be obvious flaws in the research design, or if the child is unlikely to cope well with some aspects, discuss that with the researchers. If they cannot convince you on either point, feel free to decline. Science may need altruistic volunteers to advance its frontiers, but if you have serious misgivings you are perfectly free to opt out, now or later. (And it is better to refuse to join in than to pull out half-way.)

The question of informed consent is not an easy one.[3] Many different views exist on the subject of how well-informed the patient should be. Indeed, for some people knowing too much can be a health hazard, producing a worsening of their disease state, or psychological problems. On the whole therefore you are likely to be told the minimum and left to ask questions if you want to know more—so take your time and think about it. If you do want to know more, ask open-ended questions like 'Are there other minor risks that haven't been mentioned?' 'What are the side effects of this medication?' and so on. A patient-oriented doctor will not object to such questions and will answer them fully. However, if you prefer not to know too much, the minimum may be enough. Once again, it is your decision, your responsibility. What is psychologically essential for one person may create enormous anxiety in another—so don't be persuaded (even by me) to do more or less than you feel comfortable with.

WHY IS IT SOMETIMES SO DIFFICULT TO GET MEDICAL HELP?

Some parents cannot afford the time or money to consult specialists, most of whom are in major cities. Testing is expensive and not always available on the NHS. But the basic problem goes deeper.

Medical treatments

Parents need to know that allergy and intolerance have had a very chequered career in Western medicine to date. Briefly, doctors once virtually took it for granted that what people ate or breathed had a large impact on their health, and diagnoses of 'allergy'—very imperfectly understood even by today's imperfect standards—were commonplace. But as newer schools of thought—like the psychological explanations of the effects of stress, etc.—superseded that, allergy became 'old hat'. Someone has asserted that Freud was the greatest disaster in the history of Western medicine, as he distracted everyone's attention from the biochemical basis of disease. Unfortunately, there are still those who want to explain everything they do not want to believe as being due to psychosomatic causes or placebo effects. Both are real. Neither explains a child who wakes out of a sound sleep with intense pain after being exposed—unknown to himself or his parents—to hidden foods.

Allergists did not produce 'scientific' justification of their work. (Not enough was known of the basic mechanisms to make this possible in many cases. Because of the endless variations of total body load and current tolerance level, symptoms could not always be reliably reproduced.) Allergy fell into disrepute with more 'objective' specialities within the UK (and by extension, Australian) medical world. Fortunately the clinicians continued to work in the USA and a few brave professionals in Britain and Australia continued to assert the importance of allergic, non-infective, causes of disease. As a result, even the US medical profession is deeply divided on some of these questions of 'allergy'—there are two major organizations representing different schools of thought.

The expansion of immunology led to changed terminology, which at first meant that the diagnosis of (strict) allergy was less often made, while the newer concepts of food and inhalant intolerance were not yet widely appreciated. At the present moment virtually every speciality, including allergy, is divided on the subject of the importance of diet in disease. Yet the upsurge of interest in nutrition, neurobiology and neurochemistry, endocrinology, and immunology are all moving Western medicine towards a better understanding of all this, and Britain is fortunate to have many excellent researchers in this area. It will take time to filter through to the level of the overworked GP who has not much time to read, and who is expected to be expert on everything from angina to zoster. So be patient and do not expect miracles or get angry. It does no good, where quiet persistence might.

There is a second reason for this difficulty. It is that many of the ideas now coming forward as valid or promising lines of research are 'old wives' tales' that practising professionals have been specifically taught were wrong; ideas which are currently 'out of fashion' medically. A good example is the quite recent 'discovery' of the link between colic in the breast-fed baby and the milk or other foods in mother's diet.[4] There are many pre-1940 references for that—but they were based almost entirely on clinical observations. Unfortunately as medicine becomes ever more complex, it becomes increasingly difficult for it to avoid being fashion-ridden. At present, the 'fashionable' explanations for crying babies are: (1) maternal tension and/or (2) infant temperament. Both explanations are undoubtedly 'true'—mothers of crying babies are tense and babies do differ markedly—but in my opinion and that of many other experienced mothers, both explanations beg the question entirely. Many mothers under appalling stresses have cheerful, contented babies; many babies' temperaments alter dramatically once they're no longer suffering from food-intolerance symptoms. If you wish to understand more of the history and politics of intolerance in Western medicine, read Robert Eagle's excellent little book, *Eating and allergy*. The latest landmark in this very political history was the publication, already referred to, of the Royal College of Physicians/British Nutrition Foundation Joint Report, *Food intolerance and food aversion* in April 1984. Because this is such an important document, it is discussed in some detail on p. 184 and frequently referred to.

Not all parents will be referred to an interested and informed allergist. It is perfectly possible to decide for oneself, following the simple procedures in very many self-help books. Professor Rapp's *Allergies and the hyperactive child* is one of the best of these. What is contained in this book should be sufficient to enable an intelligent parent to be reasonably sure one way or the other. Check the symptoms, try the diet diary, and so on, but only after reading enough to be sure that you appreciate the hazards. If you can, do this with the support and involvement of your doctor. The doctor who takes the time to learn about all this can be as useful as any specialist in the usual minor cases.

Medical treatments

WHAT TREATMENT IS POSSIBLE FOR FOOD AND
INHALANT INTOLERANCES?

Here there are some very different schools of thought. One school
is that of the accredited allergists and other orthodox practitioners,
including some excellent GPs. After testing to identify allergens,
the patient will be counselled to avoid known problems where this
is possible, and will be prescribed drugs where symptoms are severe
and avoidance impracticable. Some allergists will also attempt to
desensitize the patient by means of tiny, constantly increasing challenges with the allergens. Other allergists who have used sublingual (under the tongue) drops in testing, may make up drops of the
'switch-off' dosage of individual antigens, and these may effectively suppress symptoms in some people. (Although I must say
that while sublingual testing helped to identify our son's sensitivities, the drops seemed quite useless as treatment. Diagnosti-
cally they *were* useful: we had not suspected Dacron, for instance,
yet when we changed to wool pillows all nosebleeds and headaches
stopped. Accidental re-exposure brought them back.) This
approach is largely rejected by orthodox specialists,[1] though some
patients find it helpful.

Some gastroenterologists dealing with children with gut symptoms, where constant growth is important, may advocate constant
exposure of the child to amounts just below that which cause gross,
overt symptoms. (The mother usually is aware of behavioural
problems when this happens, but when the child's life is threatened
these seem bearable.) Other gastroenterologists counsel avoidance, or reduction of proven allergens. So do many thoracic
specialists dealing with asthmatics—perhaps because asthma can
kill a child far more quickly than diarrhoea. But these differences
do reflect different theories as to whether the immune response can
be induced to function better and by what means—a debate that is
far from settled.

Among orthodox practitioners, awareness of the possible importance of dietary factors has been growing. Well-designed scientific
studies, such as that of Professor Soothill's London team on migraine,[5] have made it impossible for any but the diehard to dispute
that food may cause such diverse symptoms as migraine, 'abdominal pain, behaviour disorder, fits, asthma, and eczema'. Surely this
must mean that dietary investigations will precede blanket drug

prescription? It would seem like commonsense to discover basic causes—including food and chemical sensitivities—rather than to go on prescribing drugs which suppress or alleviate symptoms. It is also cheaper for the nation as a whole, as symptomatic medication for conditions like asthma and eczema are a substantial part of Western drug budgets.

However, this sort of careful dietary investigation may not be readily available for years, even if the specialist knows that it is effective. There is a curious logic at work, expressed openly at specialist meetings, but rarely to patients. The process of testing is long, complicated and tedious for both doctor and patient alike. Compliance with the diets can be very poor, and misunderstandings common initially (how many patients 'go off milk' and never consider margarine, bread, processed foods, or even cheese as sources of milk protein?) Re-adjusting to an altered diet is difficult, and patients complain of the problems they encounter finding milk- or egg-free foodstuffs. If the doctor asks, naturally patients tell him that this change of diet causes all sorts of problems—physical, financial, social. Hence doctors are now saying to one another—'Yes, this dietary investigation works, but it's so difficult that we need to keep it *only* for the intractable or severe cases who don't respond to simple safe drugs like Intal or Ventolin.' In effect, *they* will decide whether to offer the patient this particular type of investigation and treatment; and in general they would rather continue with symptomatic treatment, whatever its costs, because it seems easier for patients and doctor alike—and more possible given an overburdened National Health Service, and the financial problems of disadvantaged families affected by the recession.

No-one would deny the difficulties inherent in careful dietary investigation and control, least of all someone like myself who has been through it with a child. However, it seems to me that such decisions must be taken by the parents, and that all options should be made known both initially and later on. I have seen families who obviously could not contemplate radical dietary change at one time, but who have grown into that decision after another couple of years of wheezing or itching. Other families try and fail, but then find the symptoms intolerable, seek practical help from parent groups, and succeed. In every case parents find that after some time their once-odd diet has become as familiar and manageable as

Medical treatments

their former one. They do still have problems, well-catalogued in Rippere's book,[6] but these require social change—which is perfectly possible once the need is publicly recognized, even if unlikely to happen overnight! So parents need to be aware that drugs remain the first choice of many orthodox practitioners. If you prefer to prevent reactions rather than to suppress symptoms—which I believe to be the more prudent course—then you may have to put some effort into convincing your doctor to refer you. You could also try convincing your MP that Britain needs more of this sort of preventive medicine. Such basic care will eventually lead to less of the highly expensive (but glamorous) medicine which threatens to bankrupt Western societies. Doctors must learn that they cannot reserve to themselves the right to decide who could cope with what type of treatment. They may be aware of the difficulties involved in such investigations, but they may not be aware of the enormous difficulties being caused by what they regard as 'minor' symptoms. Child abuse, marital breakdown, psychological damage to family members, isolation of families in society, and job loss also have social price tickets, even if we rarely quantify them in the health budget.

It is only fitting therefore, that with such issues at stake, it should be the informed patient who decides which avenue he wishes to pursue. Drugs may be necessary for an irrational and disturbed toddler—or the toddler may be eminently reasonable and willing to give up favourite foods to see if his nasty pain can be fixed. (And let us not underestimate the rationality of children who suffer symptoms from foods.) Doctors should not presume to know which course is possible or desirable unless they know the family interactions very well indeed. They should not generalize from their own family experience and expectations: doctors sometimes have problems which parents with less-demanding occupations do not, and doctors' wives can be under greater strain than other mothers for that reason alone. From observing friends, I would guess that many young doctors spend less time than average with their very young children, and are actively protected by their wives from the traumas of parenting—you cannot walk the baby for three hours at night if you may be called out to an accident or birth. Doctor fathers may well have an unrealistic idea of both normal and usual infant behaviour and the strains it imposes—they can always leave to do other things when all is chaos. (According to doctors' wives, they often do.) We non-doctors may well prove to be the real experts on children. We therefore need to know of all the options before making a choice of preferred treatment.

A second approach is that of the orthomolecular specialist. The basic underlying idea behind orthomolecular medicine is that very many people, owing to inherent deficiencies or external stresses, require far more of particular nutrients than others—and that in the absence of such supplementation, they will function at less than full capacity. Their immune system will be impaired, so that they will have more problems, both with infective illnesses and allergic disease. Many, too, have been accumulating toxins which affect bodily functioning. In short, they believe that our bodies are unbalanced; that we can find out in what ways they are unbalanced; and that attention to diet, environment, and supplementation, can put us right.[7] This all sounds commonsense and there is much to support such ideas in the work of 'conventional' nutritionists, physicians, and neurobiologists. What is more, it obviously does work for some parents—and I am certain that this is not simply a matter of placebo response in at least some cases. Equally clearly, it does not work for everyone.

But there are problems—largely to do with our ignorance of the intricate interactions between nutrients in our bodies. The orthomolecular discipline is 'new'; a lot of the treatment procedures are still experimental. Sometimes high doses are more effective than low doses—but nutrients given in high doses may be as potentially dangerous as drugs: our bodies have not evolved to be adapted to such doses. (Though human bodies are incredibly adaptable.) Sometimes low doses are more effective than high doses because they do not trigger any shut-off by the body. Sometimes nutrients given to remedy one deficiency may cause another. Sometimes they interact unexpectedly; sometimes they interact with foods and become either unavailable or excessively available. It is a very complicated business, and I doubt that many specialists would consider that they knew for certain just how vitamin, mineral, and trace element supplementation does affect each patient. And, of course, as with drugs, there is the question of the long-term impact of such treatments. Obviously this is not a do-it-yourself area of self-help, although many parents have reported that simple measures such as an increase in the B complex vitamins

Medical treatments

(not just a single B vitamin, or a few) and vitamin C have helped their family—and there is probably no real harm in trying supplementation on a small scale. Both B and C vitamins are water-soluble and readily excreted if not needed by the body. Women taking oral contraceptives should not take 1 gram or more of vitamin C, as it intensifies the many effects of the synthetic hormones. And anyone taking that amount of a synthetic vitamin supplement ought to be very careful to increase their water intake so as to prevent kidney problems, especially if taking ascorbic acid or sodium ascorbate.

The orthomolecular doctor therefore tests each individual patient to find out what possible vitamin, mineral, and trace element deficiencies may exist—and also what excesses of, for example, heavy metals such as lead, cadmium, etc. are present. Such testing is obviously necessary if an individual optimal diet and supplement is to be worked out; and the specialist is as aware as anyone could be of the interactions between nutrients. However, as with most pathology tests, this can be very expensive, and there is no guarantee that it will be of the slightest benefit to you. So parents may need to check the state of their finances, or talk it over with the doctor himself, before trying this course of action. One thing not to do is to start swallowing masses of pills without the faintest idea of whether you are deficient in anything. As with any other pills and potions, what is not necessary may do great harm.

A third school of thought is that of the clinical ecologists. This is another 'new' specialty, concerned specifically with man in his environment—or 'human illness due to common foods and environmental agents', the title of a recent conference. Clinical ecologists have a great deal in common with both orthodox specialists and the orthomolecular physicians; they probably represent a midway point. Their emphasis is slightly different: where possible they stress preventive measures, try to avoid drugs and excessive supplementation, and try to create a less-hazardous human environment. They are concerned with inhalant, food and chemical excitants—which means that pure food and water, clean air, and safe home and work environments are among their chief concerns. Most advocate a rotary, diversified diet in which patients are not too frequently exposed to any one food—the antithesis of the constant exposure theory, of course, and quite a big change in

Food for thought

kitchen organization for most of us. Dr Richard Mackarness's book *Chemical victims* outlines the clinical ecology view. Again, it has certainly worked for some parents, although his views were for a long time rejected in England. Personally, I would not advise anyone to go on to a rotary diet except as a last resort: the cost in time, money, and mental energy can be incredible. However, I must admit that some families have been greatly helped by such diets, and are able to return to more normal diets after some time.

FOOD INTOLERANCE BY PROXY?

As if there were not enough obstacles in the path of finding safe and effective treatment, a handful of psychologically needy parents have created a further and extremely distressing one. So there is now a good chance that genuinely concerned parents will be thought to be manufacturing evidence to convince doctors that their child has problems.

In 1977 Professor Roy Meadows described two cases where parents had caused their children to have numerous harmful medical procedures by fabricating both a convincing history and supporting evidence.[8] These were not cases of food intolerance. Nor were the 19 cases he discussed in a 1982 article.[9] The latter article was really quite horrifying to any normal parent, and no one would quarrel with the conclusions he reached that these were indeed disturbed parents, and that doctors always needed a small degree of suspicion, although their usual practice is (and ought to be) one of 'trusting the mother and trying to help'.[10] But evidence that parents are neurotic or obsessive finds a ready audience in medical circles, so this was taken up and christened Meadow's syndrome. A *Lancet* leading article asked the question whether 'only the lack of particular knowledge of the medical system . . . prevents more florid development' of the syndrome;[11] that is, more parents would do this sort of thing if they could (which incidentally implied that ignorance was preferable, for most of the mothers involved had some nursing knowledge).

Meadow's article was an extremely good one. He pointed out that 'It was the doctors who injured the children the most' and concluded that 'In recognising that a few mothers, by extreme fabrication, lead us to harm healthy children by our management, we should also become more aware that, even when the parent and doctor have great integrity, the potential hazards of our management for children with common problems are considerable.'[12] Those who have been through bowel biopsies and the rest would heartily agree.

It was inevitable that parents who persist in seeking solutions to problems which they perceive as allergy-related should come to be classified as having the allergic form of Meadow's syndrome, although their only 'abuse' might be to maintain a child on a particular diet against medical advice. A recent article[13] has discussed 11 families for whom the researchers consider this to be the correct diagnosis. The mindset of the authors can perhaps be judged by the fact that they quoted the *Lancet* article as having stated as fact what was raised as speculation, for which there is no evidence either way.

Unfortunately we are not given enough detail in this latter article to be able to determine whether we should agree with its authors. What precisely were the dietary inconsistencies that indicated that reactions were false? Many people can tolerate a food in a certain form, amount, or interval. What exactly was the challenge protocol used? As noted earlier, this can be utterly unreliable. What are the control challenges to which patients had to have no response before being accepted as reacting to challenge? What is meant by a 'consistent reaction from history'[14] when it is indeed 'generally known that some patients can tolerate modest quantities of particular foods if they are taken at spaced intervals but have symptoms if the same food is eaten in large quantities on consecutive days.'[15]

Obviously some of these parents had problems; although, as described, few sounded really abnormal, and none were accused of manufacturing evidence to prolong their hospital contact. Nearly half the mothers became angry and left. None of these mothers is described as seeming to enjoy their hospital stays, or being less worried about their children than the doctors, or creating close and helpful contacts with staff (all features of the Meadow's mothers), nor did they accept the diagnosis, when made, in anything like the same spirit. Nor were they eager to submit their children to painful investigations or to any perceived risk, if one can judge by tests refused or not done—again very different. The children's symptoms were real enough: 'Ten of the 17 children had mild atopic disorders, and the same 8 had evidence of allergy with positive skin

Food for thought

tests to inhalant allergens but not food allergens.'[16] (Not unusual; see p. 56.) As well as there is no suggestion in the article that they did not also have genuine nausea, abdominal pains, enuresis, coughs, fevers, and the rest. In other words, these children had problems not being manufactured by their mothers; their mothers had been trying to find explanations and remedies; and their natural parental concern made them desperate enough to try anything and to 'exhibit a limpet-like attachment to their children.'[17]

This latter point is worrying. After the experience of our son Philip's hospitalization—where only our insistence that he was not 'putting on' saved him from bowel re-section; where the one night we trusted the staff to call us if he needed us, the staff had ignored him for so long that he climbed out of his cot and began pushing it, drip and all, down the corridor; where nurses smoked their cigarettes and left young children crying—one thing is certain. If any child of mine is ever hospitalized again, my husband or I or some other adult the child trusts will be there 24 hours a day. If that's evidence of pathological mothering, then I'm pathological, and I hope my readers are too. Even if nurses were perfect, and doctors infallible, young children still need a trusted person present when they are experiencing pain and fear. So to read that one warning signal is 'any mother who is particularly attentive in prolonged visiting, or living in hospital with her child, and who refuses to leave her child alone in the ward even for an hour'[18] makes me angry. Once again, mothers can't win. If we visit too little, then our attachment is suspect and the child is uncared for; if we visit too much, we're trying to mould them into dependent invalids!

This limpet-like attachment is one of the few characteristics shared by Meadow's mothers and the 'allergy' mothers, once the two are compared carefully. Eight of 11 'allergy' mothers were well educated and articulate (of course, or they wouldn't have persisted that far). Involvement with fringe religions, spiritualism and parent self-help groups by some mothers proves what exactly? That they are not like the researchers, I presume. But I know of no evidence that spiritualists are more prone to fabricate illness; indeed, some fringe religions make it very difficult for the adherents to accept that they can be ill at all. Where their information about allergy had been obtained seems also to say very little about the mothers, except that most were still consulting medical practitioners rather than naturopaths. Analyses like this are useless,

Medical treatments

particularly in the absence of a control group of mothers whose children's food intolerances were confirmed. I'd guess that they too first heard of allergy from identical sources, and that they might include many articulate well-educated members of self-help groups, fringe religions and the rest. And any group of long-un-diagnosed patients is likely to include a substantial number with marital problems, and also psychological problems of iatrogenic origin.

Clearly, a few of the 'allergy' mothers had psychiatric problems. Their concern about their children did at least bring them into contact with professionals who could provide other resources for them and their children. Should we not therefore be grateful that these mothers got the idea of allergy and pursued it? Serious disturbances in mother–child relationships would produce symptoms of some sort, and they may well have been worse. Unlike Meadow's syndrome mothers, none abused their children, other than the one extremely disturbed mother who tried to avoid inhalant allergens by ridiculous measures

What is worrying about this article is the fact that we cannot judge for ourselves whether the researchers had eliminated the possibility of allergy in every case: we must take it on trust. After the work on migraine this is hard to accept. As well, this article may be used to further the idea of hysterical parents pursuing an obsession created by the media and by books like this; it is likely to lead to diminished trust between parents and doctors, as any intelligent parent knows immediately when the doctor begins thinking that the problem is pyschogenic. And most parents that I have talked to resent any such easy answers. So here I shall quote the part of the article that is least likely to be heard by people who think that food allergy is a fad: 'It must be emphasized that most patients investigated for food intolerance or allergy have genuine adverse rections to foods. We have continually been surprised by the variety and unexpected nature of responses to foods. There is no doubt that behaviour can be affected by allergic reactions. . . .'[19]

What can parents do if they suspect their doctor has reached the conclusion that because the tests prove negative, the problem must be psychological? It depends on the parent and the doctor. But my advice would be to be direct, to insist on talking it through. If you cannot reach agreement, agree to differ, but stay in touch. The doctor may discover more about testing procedures and reconsider; you may discover more about yourself or your child and be able to convince the doctor or even agree with him or her. Don't just disappear. If you do solve the problem, let the doctor know the details. If you take the doctor's advice, let him or her know the consequences, for doctors need feedback. It is infuriating to hear from parents of their dissatisfaction with treatment at some of the centres reputed to be the very best, and to know that their doctors consider that these patients are doing just fine on the diet/treatment they recommended. Perhaps we need some kind of independent review system to assess the success or otherwise, and the degree of patient satisfaction, before articles are published recommending a particular approach. To take an obvious example: the parents may accept a diagnosis of the child's problem arising from its inborn 'difficult temperament'. No further medical investigations are sought. Twelve months later the parents are separated because the father believed that the child could and should be punished for being difficult, and thought the mother hopelessly indulgent; while the mother still had a feeling that the child wasn't really well, and was both anxious and guilty that she could not discover the cause nor cope perfectly with the child's behaviour. Both father and mother believed that if only the mother had handled matters differently the child would have been 'normal'; so, clearly, did their family, friends and doctors. The mother was thus condemned to solo parenting of a child who had made her feel inadequate and a failure at her most basic role. The child's minor physical problems could include poor bowel control, night waking with joint pains and a cough, stomach pains and poor appetite, plus a tendency to upper respiratory tract infections. All could be seen as further proof of the mother's inadequacy, or simply as normal childhood problems; but all would put the mother, by now trying to support herself, under enormous stress. When she showed signs of such stress, this would be further proof that the child's problems stemmed from her!

This kind of vicious cycle is the not-uncommon result of ascribing physiological problems to psychological causes. As Meadow points out, there are hazards in doing the opposite, too. Perhaps the solution exists in acknowledging our ignorance of causes, which can be complex; assuring the parents that there may be unknown physical problems but they cannot be serious or they would have shown up in worse symptoms; acknowledging the strain that 'minor' symptoms can cause; and creating a support network to enable the parents to cope, and incidentally to sort through the interpersonal problems that may precede or stem from the child's problems. If parents are clearly hostile to the idea of psychological causation, they may be wrong or they may be right, but in either case it is counter-productive for a doctor to make such a diagnosis. Doctors have a far better chance of getting the parents to accept psychological help if they offer it as part of a programme to help parents cope with the *consequences* of the child's problems, than if they have suggested psychological problems as the cause. Help must be offered on the recipient's terms if it is to be of any use.

The other unfortunate consequence of the widespread publicity this syndrome will receive could be the further restriction of information to parents. The more mysterious the tests, the less parents know, the less chance there is that they could interfere or fabricate. Doctors have always agreed that a little knowledge is a dangerous thing. The logical corollary for me is to give *more* knowledge, up to the person's capacity and interest. The success of primary health workers and parents in other countries is an argument in favour of parents safely knowing a great deal more than they do in Britain and Australia, where medical knowledge is rationed more carefully than, say in the USA. (Compare the books by Lendon Smith and Hugh Jolly, for example, 'British' books for parents give signs but precious little detail of treatment; it's all 'see your doctor'.)

No doubt there are, and always will be, parents with problems who truly fit the Meadow's syndrome. No doubt too, some of us will get it wrong about allergy, and go in for silly extremes. But equally certain is the fact that some doctors will use this syndrome to write-off some of the difficult cases that more careful investigation would have uncovered as genuine. If that happens to you, don't be surprised, but don't be defeated either. See case history 6 (p. 182) which took years to be diagnosed properly, as did many others. PERSEVERE.

'MY DOCTOR SAYS IT'S THRUSH'

Earlier in the book (in Chapter 2) I discussed fungal infections, among others. This has now become a very popular diagnosis by doctors working with food- and chemical-sensitive patients. The use of massive doses of nystatin over long periods has become commonplace. Some long-term sufferers have experienced dramatic or substantial relief from symptoms after such treatment; in others, results have been negative or equivocal. Parents who want to know more about this idea should read Crooks' *The yeast connexion*. I do not dispute that fungal overgrowth is both likely (given the use of antibiotics and high-carbohydrate diets) and likely to cause problems (given the fascinating work of Dr C. Orian Truss,[22] which should be read by all professionals). But I am a little concerned at the way such diagnoses seem to be made, and the drastic regimens proposed. The high doses of nystatin used may be harmless—the companies assure us that almost none of the drug is absorbed, so its toxic potential is low—yet many people have problems with the capsule and the non-drug components, and they experience considerable nausea which impairs nutritional status. What is more worrying is the blanket prescription of a diet omitting or severely limiting all yeast, wheat, milk, sugars, and foods likely to be colonized with moulds. (Almost everything has minor amounts, however fresh it is.) As well, avoidance of antibiotics, hormonal contraceptives, steroid medications, and so on, is called for—although everyone would deplore the unnecessary use of such potent compounds. By doing so much all at once, one runs the risk of making life unnecessarily difficult. I have heard of such regimes suggested to the breast-feeding mothers of colicky babies, when the last case of colic I was consulted about required only the elimination of tea and coffee. I would emphasize again that there are risks in drastic dietary changes: risks of malnutrition, of non-compliance and increased maternal guilt and therefore stress, of increased sensitivity because normal tolerance drops during periods of avoidance, and challenges may cause new problems. So while many people have been helped by this approach, it must not become a first line of treatment. It may take more time to proceed slowly and cautiously testing obvious suspects, but it remains my choice any time.

That is also because I am a busy person. I cannot afford the time necessary to find, prepare, and persuade my children to eat a diet radically different from the social norm. I still remember vividly the horror I felt at the idea of omitting all dairy products from the family diet. What could I cook? What could we afford? How would the kids cope when we went anywhere? Of course I adjusted, and after a while found that to omit beef, food additives, and a few more, almost completely was no great work. But if someone had told me that I had to omit or reduce not just dairy products but also yeasts, sugars, and the rest—I simply would have given up on the idea unless my children were at death's door. My life was not meant to revolve endlessly around feeding the family.

Those of us who have lived with these problems for some time, and who think our diet is easy to manage despite its peculiarities, need to be very careful when talking to a mother to whom the idea is new. She is not helped by hearing the gory details of someone else's problems, and the incredibly inventive measures we have used. She may well be horrified and terrified by such accounts. A number of mothers who asked for help with a colicky baby and heard the full anti-thrush programme were simply depressed and guilty at having asked for help for what was a trivial problem from someone so much worse off. The request for help resulted in a mother who felt even more worthless and incompetent, which was not an improvement. Self-help groups often are begun or carried on by people who had had extreme problems which they resolved only with difficulty. This is understandable, as is their enthusiasm that all that they have learnt so painfully be appreciated. However, such people must constantly remember that this spectrum will include many people with relatively trivial problems, who need only relatively simple suggestions to enable them to cope. Similarly, doctors now convinced that thrush or other fungal infections are important etiological agents in food hypersensitivity must not over-diagnose. Dr Truss himself would not. It is clear that only patients with long-standing severe symptoms are considered likely cause of chronic yeast susceptibility. And I can think of few things more likely to prejudice the acceptance of this important factor by conventional medical science than even a few malnourished, wrongly diagnosed children.

'MY DOCTOR SAYS I'M HYPOGLYCAEMIC...'

This is another area of enormous controversy, as the RCP/BNF Joint Report makes very clear. They state bluntly that there is no real evidence that hypoglycaemia *per se* is responsible for adult or child ill-health. Yet some people have claimed to benefit from such

Food for thought

diagnoses. I would like to make a few points:

(1) Interpretation of blood sugar curves is a subject of controversy. The test is highly artificial. Are there wide variations in normal asymptomatic individuals? If so, what does your particular reading really signify?

(2) Even granted that you are hypoglycaemic—why are you? Difficulties in metabolizing sugar must be due to something. Forman considers that it is part of a wider process of intolerance, that the pancreas is simply one organ being affected by food and chemicals, and therefore malfunctioning.[23] No doubt others don't.

(3) Treating symptoms without ascertaining underlying causes sometimes is inescapable. But before anyone goes on to a difficult diet—and this is true of milk-free etc. diets too—one ought to be reasonably sure that the underlying cause cannot be detected and righted.

(4) Remember that simple lifestyle changes (see pp. 78–9), where possible, can also alter metabolic processes and are generally safer than dietary extremes.

(5) Remember to assess your progress and be as intelligently critical of this diagnosis as you might be of any more conventional ones, like feminine neurosis.

With hypoglycaemia, schizophrenia, and many other seemingly diverse support groups all getting together to discuss their problems, a curious consensus is emerging which supports the fact of food intolerance but debates whether this is primary or secondary. Time will tell, we hope!

7

Food intolerance and the family

HOW MUCH CAN A FAMILY DO UNAIDED?

There are quite a few helpful doctors about. In fact, one of the nicest parts of publishing this book has been discovering just how many open-minded, caring doctors there are, willing to listen and take us parents seriously. And in Britain the NHS ensures that every parent should be referred on to qualified specialists. Even so, given the present state of medical knowledge and attitudes, it may take some time to find a doctor who is helpful in this area; and he may not be able to meet all your needs for practical, detailed information.

However, to be realistic at this moment in history one must acknowledge that many parents will be unable to get really first-class professional help. This means that parents must bear a heavy burden of responsibility. Only they can decide, in the light of their particular circumstances, the apparent best course for their family. Money, isolation, access to further information, and social pressure, are all important variables. No-one can write a blueprint for anyone else to follow. **Guidelines must be intelligently interpreted in the light of individual circumstances.**

It sounds very difficult, but there are some things that make it easier. Among these is contact with people with similar problems. A formal or informal group enables parents to pool resources, to find families where visiting is easy and babysitting possible because each parent (or child)'s instructions are taken as matter of fact. Just to find another family where the mother is not thought crazy for refusing her child milk, or sweets, or orange juice, can be an enormous relief! Even if you are isolated, join a group like AAA (p. 193). Subscriptions are nominal, and will be waived if you are financially desperate. Even if you never get to a meeting, the Newsletter is full of useful practical information.

The second necessity is *some* professional help. Take the time to talk to your doctor—invite him to meet a few concerned parents and hear their story. Parents need to have their doctor aware of the problem as they see it. This is because:

1. The parents could be wrong: allergy is indeed 'the great masquerader'[1] and other conditions need to be ruled out. Once convinced of this as a problem, one tends to see it all the time. It is easy to overlook other causes.
2. The parents could be right—and their child will not receive correct treatment promptly unless their doctor knows beforehand that the child is indeed food-intolerant. (Try persuading a hospital not to give milk in any form to a convalescent child!)
3. Medication can be a useful crutch when used correctly and as little as possible. The only forms of anti-histamine freely available without prescription are the most dangerous ones —highly coloured and flavoured, loaded with sweeteners and preservatives.
4. Some reactions to foods and inhalants are life-threatening. In an emergency time shouldn't need to be wasted on explanations. (A Medic. Alert necklace or bracelet is a good idea if reactions are known to be severe.)
5. The doctor may prove to be both interested and informed, or willing to learn. A number of doctors have been involved in setting up patient self-help groups, as they know that they cannot spend the necessary time with every patient individually.

Apart from their doctor, parents need access to community dietitians (or paediatric dietitians). Once the child's diet has been stabilized, it should be checked by someone aware of the possibilities of minor deficiencies and interactions. The recent warning that too much fibre from whole grain products may lead to zinc deficiency is an illustration. Zinc is an important factor in adequate growth; it is needed in the formation of important body enzymes. Some growth retardation may be due not to malabsorption due to intolerance, but because of this. Of course, if the dietitian consulted insists that a child cannot be adequately fed without dairy products, as has happened, parents can choose whether to smile politely and keep looking for help, or to stay there and convince her/him. Your doctor or paediatrician can refer you to a dietitian. The British Nutrition Foundation should be able to help you find nutritionists and sources of nutritional advice. The

Food intolerance and the family

Department of Health should have copies of tables listing the contents of British foods—write and ask.

If the parent simply wants someone to sound out ideas on, the local clinic sister is sometimes a great help. (Sometimes not—but it is not difficult to know.) Some health visitors have become extremely interested and informed on this subject. Remember that there are mutual advantages in talking to the professionals—they may be unaware of these problems unless parents are confident and strong enough to tell them. From what parents have written, this seems to be a real difficulty. Parents are aware that prescribed regimes or drugs aren't working, but won't tell the doctor—especially the hospital-based specialist—because they are afraid to. Having been a patient myself, I can well understand that feeling. But it must be resisted. Doctors need to be told what works and what doesn't. It is not your role in life to 'keep doctor happy' but to co-operate in the difficult process of finding real solutions for yourself or your child. Good doctors don't want you to confirm their prejudices but to be honest with them. Being aware of the discrepancy between what patients tell me and what they tell the doctor makes me realize just how unscientific and fallible a lot of medical practice must be. So do your bit—tell them! Every case they know of makes it easier for the next family—who may be socially more disadvantaged than you. As she has access to resources denied to parents, the health visitor can be a great ally.

It might be politic, but would not be just, to omit consideration of 'alternative medicine'—the naturopaths, chiropractors, acupuncturists, homeopaths, and so on. As one reared on 'orthodox' medicine, I am aware of the partly justified, wholly emotional reaction against such 'quacks'. As a very unsusceptible patient, I am aware that some are capable of doing more in certain conditions than orthodox medicine. An increasing number of other Australians know that too. Awareness of the importance of nutrition has been a hallmark of alternative medicine. I suspect that within another few decades, orthodox and alternative medicine will be engaged in more fruitful dialogue.

For the present though, there are problems. Standards of training and expertise are very variable in those disciplines not subject to any external regulation. (Mind you, that is not untrue of orthodox medicine either.) 'Prescriptions' can be as obscure and dogmatic as any old style medic. And as has already been stated, overdoses of nutrients are as pharmacologically active and potentially dangerous as any 'synthetic' drug. Spinal X-rays and manipulation can also be dangerous in unskilled hands. So it undoubtedly pays to be a critical consumer where any medicine, orthodox or alternative, is concerned. Too often parents don't ask for explanations or raise questions; they don't understand the proposed treatment and yet don't query it. They don't ask the age and dosage of the X-ray machine and decline to be subjected to unnecessary radiation. They should!

Still it must be said—chiropractors, naturopaths, homeopaths, and the like have helped many families more than their previous orthodox consultants. This is *not* all placebo effects: infant eczema or other symptoms are not easily influenced by maternal faith, or othodox doctors would have a better cure rate! Most parents have been influenced by the medical attitude of mistrust—they go to alternative practitioners in fear and trembling, as a last resort; whereas they approach their family doctor—initially at least—with an unbounded confidence in his almost godlike knowledge. (A silly attitude which is responsible for a lot of unnecessary pressure on doctors; it makes it almost impossible to admit to not knowing something.)

Having said all that, what can parents do totally unaided—in the outback perhaps, or when they can afford neither orthodox nor alternative medicine, and public hospital facilities collapse for lack of funding? What follows in Part Two is meant to answer that question. Ideally it is not a substitute for professional help but a preliminary to it. Remember too that, while there are dangers in being without medical and nutritional supervision when experimenting with diet, there are also dangers in ignoring the problem. Parents and children alike have only one unique and irreplaceable body.

Other simple things you can do without hesitation include:

- Regular exercise, which has all round health benefits but which is also said to stimulate the immune system.[2]
- Stress-control techniques. Simple breathing and meditation exercises all the way through to biofeedback are increasingly recognized as helpful to parents and children alike.
- Avoid *elective* surgery in the first few years of life. That includes circumcision of course. An article in a recent

78

paediatric journal demonstrated that the white blood cells of stressed newborn infants had decreased bacteria—killing power.[3] In a previous issue another author had argued that the avoidance of elective surgery . . . may significantly lessen the likelihood of major respiratory allergies.[4]

- Overall good diet, which everyone now seems to agree is low-fat, low-salt, high-fibre, less meat, more fruit, vegetables, and whole grain cereals. As a recent BBC documentary pointed out, that is what the 'faddists' had been saying for forty years before it was 'scientifically proved'.
- Massage. Marvellous for parents and children alike. If it can be combined with acupressure by a knowledgeable practitioner, or better still, acupuncture, it may be of even greater benefit. (That, too, is gradually becoming respectable after years of condemnation.)

If you are generally healthy, fit and unstressed, your body is more likely to be able to cope with both allergic and infectious challenges.

SOME OTHER INTERESTING IDEAS TO CONSIDER

Some other interesting ideas have emerged from such diverse groups as hyperactive children, schizophrenics, and multiple sclerosis victims. Some parents have found that the addition of zinc and/or digestive enzymes to the diet improved the child's stools and growth, and with that improvement came a decrease in intolerance symptoms. This points up once again the importance of good nutritional status—in making sure that the child is receiving enough essential amino acids and other nutrients for its immune system to work efficiently. Other parents found that an increase in protein intake (not all at once but spread over the day) also improved growth and symptoms. Here perhaps I should say that while vegetarian diets can be first rate, there is no room for casualness when breast-feeding or feeding a child on a vegetarian, especially a vegan diet. Recent reports of brain damage due to B vitamin deficiencies, and other tragedies, make it imperative that vegetarian diets are very carefully worked out to provide sufficient essential amino acids, fatty acids, and other nutrients. Consult a nutritionist, and read the books by Frances Moore Lappé as a beginning.

Food for thought

Too much digestive enzyme added to the diet might cause serious problems, perhaps by damaging stomach lining, or by decreasing the body's already inadequate secretion of such enzymes—any body system not being used tends to atrophy. Too much protein might lead to damaging levels of breakdown products in the body, and to further sensitivity. So these are ideas to be discussed with your doctor and nutritionist, and cautiously tested.

A third line of action comes from Bristol eczema researchers[5] and multiple sclerosis self-help groups[6]—supplementation with certain essential fatty acids. This I find particularly interesting. When I first learnt of the gulf between breast and bottle in the matter of fatty acid composition, and knew that essential fatty acids were required for the myelination of the brain and central nervous system, I could not help asking whether diseases due to defects in myelin were not becoming more common wherever breast-feeding had been abandoned. Perhaps not surprisingly I discovered that is exactly what is happening. Yet in the discussion of the geographical distribution of multiple sclerosis, I have never seen this possibility raised. Of course it is likely to be only one factor, with later childhood and adult diet just as important—but it surely cannot help to start out in life deficient in some essential fatty acids, and perhaps lacking some altogether. It has now been shown that the composition of infant body fat is heavily dependent on diet, and the fatty acid composition of breast milk varies with maternal diet as well as infant age. (No recommendations about maternal diet have followed, but it would seem sensible for mothers to make sure that their diet contains good sources of polyunsaturated fats, especially certain essential fatty acids. Polyunsaturated fats include sunflower and safflower seed oils, preferably cold-pressed. These can be blended with butter to produce a spread that tastes better than commercial margarines, reduces the butter-addict's saturated fat intake, and is free of added chemicals. Nutritionists tend to suggest using margarines, but I have never liked the idea since reading that at one stage of manufacture the product is a black sludge. Butter in small quantities seems vastly preferable. Other nutritionists urge us to use *no* fatty spreads on our bread, which is more logical, since we take in enough from other food sources anyway.)

Does essential fatty acid supplementation help in food intolerance? Trials with evening primrose oil in eczema patients suggest

Food intelligence and the family

so, and the RCP/BNF Report stated that such supplementation 'may be more appropriate than dietary restriction.'[7] There is not room to argue the case, but essential fatty acids of the linolenic and linoleic families are needed not only for myelin, but in the formation of prostaglandins, chemicals involved in the immune response. Zinc, and vitamins B and C, are also needed in prostaglandin synthesis—and these are the nutrients most commonly found to be useful supplements by allergic families. This is a very new and exciting area—but don't rush out and experiment! As always, there are hazards. This has been extremely well discussed in a very readable book by Judy Graham (see p. 219). It was interesting to see how prominently food intolerances also featured in her book and how compatible the dietary advice given is with what 'allergy' victims are told. Of course the suggestions given for people with established multiple sclerosis are probably excessive for those of us whose problems are less severe and I disagree about some aspects of allergy testing. None the less I think everyone ought to read this book—or everyone who intends changing the family diet, at least!

SOME FEELINGS PARENTS MUST COPE WITH IN ALL THIS

1. Guilt

Most parents and grandparents after putting together the jigsaw pieces of their child's problems, realize that their actions have been an important contributing cause. Some feel very guilty that they:

— food-binged in pregnancy
— did not breast-feed
— did not breast-feed long enough
— allowed 'comps', or gave them
— introduced solids early
— punished their children for lack of bladder or bowel control
— became angry over tantrums, etc.
— did not believe their child's account of feeling ill
— forced children to eat certain foods
— smoked while pregnant or with children, or were addicted to coffee, or whatever

and so on and on. All of those things are certainly cause for regret, even for open acknowledgement to the children themselves. But guilt is an inappropriate response. There are two things for parents to remember:

1. **None of it is your fault,** provided you tried to do the best for your kids—as we all do—most of the time. In any case, you cannot be *sure* that what you did was the major cause of the problem that developed: it could have happened that way whatever you did, or might even have been worse!

2. **You are the victims,** as much as your children; victims of the social attitudes and practices that still say to most people that nutrition isn't important, that the bottle is 'just as good', that breast-feeding 'isn't nice', or whatever. In such a case, guilt is a waste of energy.

Apart from regret, the emotion parents would be justified in feeling is not guilt, but anger. Take the whole issue of breast-feeding. Who should feel guilty about that? Not the mothers, atlhough the observation that many will, and do, is used as a reason to keep silent about the problems of bottle-feeding. Would those mothers feel guilty if they knew that probably 95 per cent of women could successfully breast-feed if motivated (by hard information, not sentimental appeals), well managed in hospital, and supported at home? I suspect that women might feel cheated, and angry. That fewer than this do breast-feed, and that almost no baby escapes the bottle, is an indictment of our 'health-care' system. There could be few simpler, cheaper, more cost-effective pieces of preventive medicine than the education and care of pregnant and lactating mothers—yet the majority who succeed at breast-feeding currently do so almost *despite* our hospitals and doctors. If you 'failed', it was probably because others failed you.

In every species there will be some who have difficulty adequately feeding their offspring. But in our ingenious society, it should be perfectly possible for those babies to receive human milk for their first 6 months. The enormous resources that have gone into modifying cows' milk are a testimony to what can be done. Human mothers are in fact more efficient milk producers than cows, believe it or not, and I would hope that we'd have less bacterial contamination than the average udder! Maybe it's time for the wet-nurse to make a comeback?. . . If we are interested in child health, and in long-term adult health, we may need to adjust our cultural mindset, and shed a few prejudices.[8] Of course, this is impractical, a counsel of perfection, at present. No-one realizes that more keenly than I do. But unless an ideal is stated, there is no impetus to change a far from ideal situation.

We could look at almost every issue related to diet and environment in the same way. Certainly informed parents would do things differently—but whose responsibility is it that parents are not informed? One could hardly say that mass advertising and the mass media, which reach every family, are entirely blameless. In a consumer society, community education and preventive health are very low priorities—they are not growth industries. Sickness is, and so is poor nutrition. But who gains if all women breast-feed? Formula manufacturers, the dairy industry, the medical professions, the advertising companies and so the media, the drug companies, the hospitals all lose. (Babies gain, but they don't vote or spend money.) Is it surprising that the UK does not intend to enact legislation to enforce the WHO Code of Marketing of Breastmilk Substitutes; that instead an industry code has been accepted; that hospitals are littered with industry-promotional material; and so on and on? No-one would argue that this is all a deliberate plot by wicked or stupid people—though greed, institutionalized in our way of life, is a large part of the explanation. Such short-sightedness is simply the inevitable result when the interests of the powerful coincide, and those who seek change are the powerless. Self-interest can make fools of us all. Still feeling guilty?

2. Depression

Unlike guilt, there are good reasons to feel daunted, depressed, or very switched-off about all this. It seems as though the more you know, the worse it all gets—more complicated, more decisions to make, and so on. What should be a simple pleasure becomes one great hassle. Some people react by saying that they just do not want to know about it—this is usually the busy mother who realizes with sinking heart that she will have to rethink everything from shopping to cooking to parties, etc. It is also, often, the unaware addict who simply cannot imagine coping without his/her coffee, cigarettes, milk, chocolate, sugar, raw lemons, or coke (loaded with caffeine).

Food for thought

There is some good news to be stated here.

- Firstly, it is *not* as bad as you would expect (unless yours is a severe case). Thinking about it is often the worst part.
- Secondly, the benefits outweigh the hassles—*especially* if yours is a severe case—and are often surprising.
- Thirdly, no-one is telling you that you *must* do this—you can decide for yourself whether it is worth the effort and no-one can or should dispute that decision.
- Fourthly, it has its uses. Many mothers find that it solves the social problem of junk food—the child knows he cannot have it or he hurts; the mother can say that it's for medical reasons that she will not allow it, not because she is mean or moralistic or thinks herself better than those mums whose kids seem to live on flavoured milk, ice lollies, and chips.

But playing Pollyanna can only go so far. This whole business does put the burden of responsibility for our health, and our children's, squarely on our own shoulders. It makes us aware of the fact that we do only have one body, and that what we do with it matters. Certain specialists are afraid that this sort of knowledge could create an epidemic of hypochondriacs—people obsessed with anxiety about their health. Commonsense has to come in here again—we do what we can, within the limits of what we can learn, and after that we live with it. An awareness of what we do should not necessarily mean neurosis. In any case, there seems no shortage of neurosis among those who pay no attention to diet and health.

And when it does seem too much—find another parent and compare notes. Sometimes there are very simple solutions to current problems; sometimes depression in itself a symptom. Sometimes you need to have a cry.

3. Anger

Although I have suggested that this is an appropriate human response, it's not a particularly fair or useful one and needs to be channelled constructively. After all, the particular people with whom you are angry—often for good reason—are as they are because of their education and life experiences, for which they too are not wholly responsible. It always pays to try to find out why

Food intolerance and the family

such people think and act as they do. Try to talk with them; if that fails try to write a clear statement of your position (keep a carbon); if that fails, go elsewhere. But use some of the steam generated to stir some movement for change. There is a great deal that any one of us can do.

4. Frustration and disappointment

These are possible companions. Some people identify their problem foods and hey presto! nothing further to worry about. Other people find it incredibly difficult to discover/avoid problem substances; others may have everything under control and then it's suddenly downhill again. To be disappointed over a child's sudden regression, or frustrated with any number of things, is all too common. Some mothers come close to despair at times. Learn from your experience, talk to other parents and learn from theirs. It all sounds terribly trite, but it is true. This may just be something you have to accept. Techniques of stress control, such as relaxation exercises, may help you cope, and many doctors now prescribe a tape rather than an anti-depressant.

5. Anxiety

There are times for all of us when we fervently wish we had never heard about any of this. We worry that what we are doing is right or harmful, about the long-term consequences, and so on. Indeed, that is a reason, advanced by a minority of professionals, for not educating parents; it will only serve to raise maternal anxiety levels, which certainly isn't a good thing.

Individuals are all very different. Some people are anxious when they know too little, others when they know too much. A degree of anxiety is both normal and inevitable for parents—who could escape it with all the social, economic, political, chemical, and military threats that cloud our children's future? One simply has to face facts, do the best one can, and then find alternative ways of discharging anxiety. (Some will escape into a book, others into a bout of spring-cleaning—it doesn't matter what method you use.) You will be anxious—of course. But you would have been anxious anyway, if your child kept on being ill, or disagreeable, or wakeful, or whatever. At least this gives you a 'no-fault' explanation to hang on to—you don't have to be anxious over whether it's your parenting or her personality—it's a problem external to you both. Hang

85

Food for thought

on to that and try to avoid the anxiety drugs, with their many side effects. (Did anyone ever tell you that they affect memory, for instance?) And on the whole, the real options and possibilities you are anxious about are less horrendous than the possibilities you imagine in the absence of reliable information—or so I find!

SOME SPECIAL EFFECTS IN WOMEN

Some curious observations have emerged from the families that have been followed up. There seems to be a definite, hormone-linked variation in the degree to which a woman's gut is affected by food excitants, and so the degree to which her breast-fed baby is affected. Women had noticed that their breast-fed babies screamed and/or refused the breast in the few days before a period; this changed with dietary changes. Women who had suffered severe premenstrual tension (PMT), or migraines, also noted improvement. These women were also given to recurrent or chronic mastitis for which no traumatic cause was found, and they bruised easily. This all seems to suggest that their antigen uptake was greater at such times, and that this higher antigen load (or perhaps their prostaglandin levels) was affecting their vascular system[9] perhaps allowing the passage of immune complexes into breast or brain tissue, with subsequent inflammation etc. Women who note the correlation of PMT, migraine, bruising, and mastitis may thus do well to identify the foods to which they are susceptible, and to see if this 'vascular syndrome' improves. Alcohol would probably affect this, through its action on smooth muscle and blood-vessels. The effect of oral contraceptives also needs investigation—some women found them to cause severe migraine. And although this is hotly refuted by many researchers who say, once again that there is no scientific proof, breast-feeding mothers in Australia, USA and the UK report that oral contraceptives sometimes cause irritability on the breast-fed baby, depress the milk supply, and are linked with maternal depression as well.[10] Probably thousands of women can safely use a very-low-dose Pill while breast-feeding—but the observation that many mothers and babies are affected seems universal. Barrier methods would seem to be the more appropriate choice while breast-feeding, although each couple must decide in the light of their own circumstances, of course.

86

Food intolerance and the family

Another comment women frequently make is that their capacity to cope with certain foods was much greater before becoming pregnant. Many have found tea, coffee, milk, or other foods nauseating and their sensitivity to alcohol much greater, in pregnancy. Many of these find that even after childbirth they cannot tolerate such items. Some find it hard to adjust to the altered reality of their bodies (in this as in other ways) and push themselves to return to 'normal'. Maybe we women have to accept that childbearing creates a new normal for some of us.

The above observations were all noted in 1982, and at that time I could find very little medical support for them, though they were indubitably true. Naturally I was delighted to find the RCP/BNF Joint Report noting that 'women patients sometimes say they can drink wine but not during their premenstrual week, or that their migraine disappears during pregnancy and is exacerbated by the contraceptive pill.'[11] Perhaps women will be taken seriously now, when they comment on these effects.

8

Drugs and their action

Because of the complicated nature of the allergic response, it is possible to block its effects at different points by different chemicals. Many books discuss the relevant drugs. I only want to mention those available without prescription. (Doctors should tell their patients about those they prescribe. If they don't have time to, ask your chemist to let you read the relevant pieces in MIMS, Martindale, or the *British National Formulary* and explain them to you.)

Drugs, being potent chemicals, no parent should give medication without good cause. This is especially true for intolerant children, as they are at risk of reacting not only to the drug, but also to the fillers, preservatives, etc. Lactose is quite commonly used, for instance, and commercial-grade lactose is contaminated with milk protein. Corn derivatives are also common at present. However, the *Pediatrics* advertisement gives some hope that commercial drug companies are becoming aware of these problems, at least in America.

That being said, it would be inhumane to refuse relief to the child who wakes crying with pain. Anti-histamines and anti-inflammatory drugs are both available and can help.

ANTI-HISTAMINES

These include promethazine, available in syrup form. There are a wide variety of anti-histamines available on prescription. In dealing with a young child, only the syrups permit the precise tiny dosage to be accurately measured. But once the child is big enough to swallow a tablet, or part of one, parents should ask the doctor for non-coloured, non-sweetened tablets. They can be cut to size—carefully, and if necessary crushed in water with perhaps a little honey, maple syrup, or other tolerated sweetener.

These drugs are often prescribed for 'cold' symptoms. But children sometimes respond unexpectedly to them. Some children become excessively sleepy, and others become unnaturally active.

Drugs and their action

Many children who are neither feel fairly woolly-headed, grumpy, and even head-achey next day, especially if the medication was given late during the night. It pays to think about the timing of anti-histamines—if the child can sleep it off overnight he will probably be OK. (The idea of children taking antihistamines for months every year is simply appalling.)

ANALGESICS

Aspirin and paracetamol are the two most common analgesic (pain-killing) and anti-inflammatory drugs available without a prescription. There have been many reported cases of hypersensitivity to aspirin, especially in the child who is sensitive to salicylate-containing foods. I am not aware of any such reported reactions to paracetamol. For this reason it is possibly safer to give the child the appropriate dose of paracetamol. Again, use the syrups as little as possible; tablets can be cut up carefully, crushed and dissolved in water. Some children respond better to the soluble forms of paracetamol.

All these drugs are thought of as 'safe'. They are, in some sense that adverse effects are minimal and infrequent *provided instructions are followed*. They are not, in the sense that an overdose could easily cause drastic harm and that no-one can entirely predict how a small body will react to them. The less attractive they are to the children—the more awful the taste—the less chance there is that your child will swallow the bottle on the odd occasion when you forget and leave it about. For medication to be a delicious treat is hardly very sensible. Our parents managed to get the most obnoxious tasting mixtures into us without profound psychological harm resulting—why are we so hesitant? Of course the kid won't like it, but you'll both survive the ordeal.

Analgesics usually have no hang-over effect, and can be given at any time of day. By reducing inflammation and pain, they do help the child ride out the painful reaction. If your child seems to have an adverse reaction, write to the company who made the drug and find out *exactly* what is in it. Record this in his medical history. If the company won't tell you, send the correspondence to the Consumers' Association, or the Society for Environmental Therapy (p. 196).

Food for thought

Probably rate a mention here. Some contain drugs which help to relieve muscle spasm in the gut—which should help. But all contain alcohol, a potent smooth-muscle relaxant. It is quite possibly the alcohol which helps baby's gut stop spasming; grandma's a 'few drops of brandy in warm water' was possibly just as good. However, alcohol is a central nervous system depressant—and thus would not be a good idea in young babies with immature breathing patterns. The withdrawal of some of these drugs from the market strengthens my concern about drug use in children. One manufacturer now states that they should not be given to infants under 6 months, so they are no longer 'colic' remedies.

If your child has shown any sensitivity to any drugs, this should be recorded in his Medic-Alert bracelet. Be careful to mention the fact of his food or drug reactions *to the anaesthetist on the day of any operation*, however minor—if the anaesthetist knows the child is sensitive and has been reminded just before surgery, he will be extra-vigilant and may even use different drugs. Difficulty with anaesthetics is not a rare occurrence in these children.[10]

9

Some unanswered questions

Many basic questions seem unanswered. Some of particular interest to parents include:

(1) Whether
   (i) circadian rhythms
   (ii) menstrual cycle and other hormonal changes
   (iii) physical exercise
   have any effect on antigen uptake and secretion. Many curious observations by mothers might be explained under these headings.

(2) Whether antigens have cumulative and/or synergistic effects.

(3) Whether the physical form of the antigen is more important than quantity in determining symptoms.

(4) Whether allergens are more/less potent in
   (i) high sugar, salt, alcohol combinations
   (ii) high fibre combinations.

(5) Whether total dietary elimination leads to hypersensitivity to tiny amounts when re-exposed.

(6) Whether the gastroenterologists 'push to limits then reduce' theory *can* induce intolerance. Is this preferable to or less desirable than total avoidance? Or is reduction but NOT elimination the best course? At present, pure chance seems to determine the advice parents receive—respiratory and skin and gastrointestinal symptoms are all treated in very different ways.

(7) Whether immunological boosting/challenge—via injection—leads to better or worse immune function. (Many allergic children really had trouble after the usual childhood immunizations.) Although there are many obvious benefits of mass immunization, it seems that the food-intolerant child needs special care before and after. It

could be that many of the adverse reactions reported after injections are occurring in the unrecognized allergic child. Perhaps 2 months is too young for the fully breast-fed allergic baby?

(8) Whether expressed human milk has any therapeutic value in the older allergic child or adult. (My findings and those of the La Leche League in America suggest that it may have. Among other points, it's interesting to note that the toddler still being breast-fed instinctively tended to refuse other foods and revert to full breast-feeding in periods of illness, whether infective or allergic. Where this was allowed, the child's recovery seemed more rapid to the parent.)

(9) Why so many children develop respiratory symptoms at age 4–5.

(10) Whether the infant gut recovers completely (when foods are totally avoided) and, if so, up to what age. (It seems as though some babies, when given a long spell of exclusive breast-feeding with the mother avoiding known allergens, do recover; but the children had not been followed up for long enough to be sure that this is permanent.)

(11) Whether the use of gastric and pancreatic proteolytic enzymes before and/after eating assists the food-intolerant person.

(12) Whether parental smoking is significantly linked with the development of childhood food intolerances. (In this sample, the mothers of seriously affected children all proved to be smokers and, in some cases, were themselves the children of smokers.)

(13) What range of variation there is between mothers in their uptake and excretion of dietary antigens; and whether some mothers would be best advised to seek donated human milk while identifying their allergens.

(14) What the intolerant mother should do before conceiving another child, and in subsequent pregnancies.

(15) Whether cystitis, vaginal discharge, and other genitourinary symptoms may be the result of food intolerance.

(16) Whether children with food-intolerance problems are more likely than others to develop a limp, perhaps as the result of inflammatory joint changes.

Some unanswered questions

(17) Whether our cultural stereotypes of 'normal' child health and behaviour have been warped by our cultural experience of unrecognized food intolerance.

(18) Whether our modern epidemic of baby battering is one result of excessive crying due in many cases to food intolerance.

(19) Whether biological and psychological disturbances such as learning disabilities, schizophrenia, autism, and many others may be partly caused by food and chemical intolerance.

(20) Whether inappropriate infant nutrition is a factor in many diseases, including autoimmune diseases, diabetes, inflammatory bowel diseases, etc. *ad infinitum*. Why details of mode of infant feeding are not recorded as part of every medical history, so far as is practicable.

(21) Why govenment bodies concerned about optimal health and minimal health costs do not more actively promote to the general public the national dietary guidelines, and UNICEF's four-point campaign, while at the same time curbing the activities of those who promote foods etc. which offend against those guidelines. Why there is so little community and parent education being undertaken, despite the cost-effectiveness of such measures.

'EVERYWHERE I LOOK I SEE ALLERGY!'

There is a real danger that after a while everything will seem to fit the pattern of problems with food and inhalant intolerance. We do have to remember that there are other causes of illness and behavioural problems. But in one way we're probably right to see it almost everywhere.

After all, we each have only one body, with all its parts interacting. The relationship between infectious disease and an over-taxed immune system is easily seen. Health represents a state in which our bodies are coping well with all the stresses we expose them to—bacterial and viral challenge, fatigue, psychologically induced hormonal change, and so on. Food is the foreign object that we bring into closest proximity to our bodies—only the lining of our digestive system separates it from our body tissue. It is hardly surprising that on occasions, perhaps in everyone's life, enough of

93

Food for thought

it breaches the body's defences to cause minor or major disturbances. Seen from this perspective, it seems ridiculous that anyone
can accept that drugs and chemicals can cause problems, but that
the chemicals we call 'food' should not. Why not?

Remember, too, the impact of changing food habits. Glaser, like
Hambraeus, sees the substitution of cows' milk for human milk in
infancy as an uncontrolled experiment; he sees it as responsible for
'the apparent rapid increase in the development of the allergic
diseases over the past 30–40 years'.[1] Where once 'allergy' was
though to affect perhaps 6–7 per cent of the population, the US
figures now range from 28–35 per cent.[2] (That of course is only
major disease—asthma and eczema chiefly). Other social habits,
like forcing children to eat food which repelled them, and to eat up
everything on the plate, were possibly also instrumental in producing gut damage that we as parents still suffer from—and that our
children suffered from in the womb and while being breast-fed.

So if, like me, you are really anxious to meet someone who has
definitely not been affected at all by this food-intolerance business,
and if such people seem hard to find, take refuge in the thought
that major dietary revolutions might be expected to produce major
social effects. Remember the Japanese after the Second World
War—the Americanization of their diet has meant that buildings
and transport vehicles have all had to be enlarged as Japanese
children grow up and tower over their parents. No-one really fore-
saw that at the time, either.

However, what is done is done. There is not much point in
recriminations, since we would have done much the same had we
been a product of those times. Let us concentrate on what can be done
here and now to improve the lot of food-intolerant families.

AN APPEAL TO VESTED INTERESTS

If you are a dairy farmer, obviously you will not like to see parents
taking their children off milk products without good cause. In this
current generation there are many children who would be healthier without milk, or without much milk, for most of their lives.
Economically that is disastrous if it becomes widely known. But
the remedy is in your hands. If children under 6 months or so are
not exposed to milk products or any other food than human milk,
the likelihood of severe intolerance is enormously reduced. Can

Some unanswered questions

you not join with us in getting all infants off to the best possible start, so that as hungry toddlers and schoolkids they can be given any good food, including milk? It is in your own interest. My son probably received only a litre or so of milk in his first week in hospital. Now, at 9, he cannot tolerate even the small amounts of milk powder in bread. Our family consumption of milk has dropped from 3 litres a day to a litre a week—I can't cook with milk. I know dozens of families like us. Read this book carefully—wouldn't it be in everyone's best interests, economically as well as medically, for milk to be promoted in a more discriminating way? For dairy producers to support bodies whose work helps to reduce the chances of allergy? Please let me know what you think.

And I would appeal to medical and paramedical vested interests too, to listen to parents, and to adopt an attitude of greater humility, of willingness to admit ignorance even, and willingness to learn. No-one doubts the sincerity of your desire to serve the community. But no intelligent parent expects you to be omniscient. When you refuse to listen to our observations, and offer half-baked psychological explanations that are impertinent as well as irrelevant, you forfeit our respect. When you refuse to apologize for considering us 'obsessive' or 'neurotic' until the day when we are proved incontrovertibly right to be concerned about our children—when you then pass some jocular comment or ignore the past entirely—we are disappointed in you. When you refuse to alter hospital practices that arise from outdated beliefs and attitudes, you cause us to wonder whether you think the patients exist to serve the hospital's needs, rather than the reverse.

We parents are concerned about the quality of the care and advice we have been given. We find it hard to talk back to you, for there are many ways that you can make life difficult for us if we do. We feel that if only you would try to enlist us as collaborators and allies, our care would improve and your workload be lightened. But none of it will happen unless you can learn to take us seriously, and to encourage us to use what intelligence and perception we possess. Unless you do this, you should not be surprised if the drift to alternative medicine becomes ever stronger.

We want to utilize all the best medical resources for our children. When we are driven to write books such as this—and there is an explosion of material on medical topics written by laymen—we do so in the hope that you will respond to it with

95

Food for thought

compassion, honesty, and intelligence. If you have criticisms to make, please do so—not from any lofty position of scientific precision, for we know that most of your clinical practice is not 'scientific'—but simply from the standpoint of another, perhaps better-informed human being. The god-like stance of some of the doctors of yesteryear is simply not credible for those of us who know how often accepted practice has been reversed.

Our thanks to those exceptional professionals who are pioneering this work (based as it is on a premise that the patient can be trusted to want to be well); to those doctors and nurses and others who have treated us as intelligent human beings and sought to do the best possible thing for us and our families. Please don't think us ungrateful to criticize the profession: you are the exceptions that give us hope that change is possible, and fortunately, there seem to be more of you around the world than we might have guessed!

'Food allergy has, in the past, been variously regarded as part of fringe medicine or a kind of cult subject, attracting the attention of newspapers, television, and the more popular medical journals . . . As the evidence accumulates, however, clinical reactions to food—both allergic and non-allergic—are seen to be of considerable importance . . . it is clear that people who have symptoms of food intolerance should no longer be offered a crude approach to diagnosis and a blunderbuss approach to treatment. Whether they have enzyme defects, other causes of food idiosyncracy, food allergy or psychological problems, those who react to foods . . . deserve to have their problem examined carefully.'

M.H. Lessof (ed.) *Clinical reactions to food*. Wiley, Chichester (1983), p. ix.

PART 2

Practical aids

10

Are you or your child food-intolerant?

HOW TO DECIDE

You are more likely to be if you are one of those:

— born into an intolerant family—do your relatives suffer from eczema, asthma, hayfever, etc.?
— born of a mother who smoked, drank alcohol, or food-binged in pregnancy;
— born of a mother who forced herself to eat 'good' foods that made her feel ill while pregnant or breast-feeding;
— born of a mother who had suggestive symptoms in her childhood;
— exposed to foreign protein early in infancy;
— exposed to foreign protein after diarrhoea or any abnormal gut state such as gastroenteritis;
— born of particular racial groups—e.g. Asians and others whose traditional diet doesn't include milk but who are now using it extensively;
— who dislike certain foods but who force themselves to eat those foods;
— who binge on any foods, who have cravings for particular foods, who drink lots of tea, coffee, and cola in a day, etc. After an initial stage of intolerance, the body can adapt so as to become addicted to certain foods. Elimination will lead to withdrawal symptoms. Suspect this if you 'just don't feel right' unless you have an egg for breakfast, or some other inflexible food habit;
— had any of the symptoms listed on p. 33 when an infant (consult your parents!) or have any of those that follow.

99

Food for thought

N.B. Other explanations are possible for each and all of these. A number, however, is suggestive of intolerance, especially, if accompanied by changes in temperature and pulse. (Learn what *is* your child's normal temperature and pulse rate—it is often at least ½ degree below 'average'—by measuring when he/she is well, over a period of time.)

(a) In infancy—(see p. 33)
(b) School age—as above, plus:

— learning difficulties due to short concentration span, and sometimes due to hearing difficulties which can come and go with food exposures;
— restlessness or sluggishness;
— night walking, restless sleep, sudden fevers;
— bed-wetting, stress incontinence;
— stomach pains, leg aches, night cramps, limb and joint pains—may occur anytime, but may wake child at night, or occur before school (after breakfast or on an empty stomach), joint swelling, stiffness;
— persistent night cough, coughing on exertion, constant throat-clearing;
— itchy mouth, nose, throat, or eyes; mouth ulcers;
— recurrent sinusitis, tonsillitis, pharyngolaryngitis, ear infections, rhinitis, croup;
— blinking;
— pallor, with dark rings under the eyes, easy bruising;
— headaches;
— asthma.

(c) Pre-adolescent—adulthood—as above, plus

— itchy eyes or mouth, watering eyes, photophobia (intolerance of light);
— hayfever (sensitive to pollen, dust, pollution, cigarette smoke, animals, moulds, etc.)
— chronic sinusitis;
— migraine headaches, recurrent headache;
— tension-fatigue syndrome: difficult personality, poor

100

achievement, depression, waking up more tired than when one went to bed;
— giant hives;
— food bingeing or compulsive eating
— recurrent non-infective urinary tract inflammation;
— premenstrual difficulties;
— recurrent or chronic mastitis unexplained by normal causes (see NMAA booklet, *About breast and nipple problems; NMAA Newsletter* July 1982) Available through NCT, or direct from NMAA (see p. 202);
— mental confusion, many forms of mental disorder (see Mackarness);
— tinnitus (noises in the ear);
— vertigo (giddiness);
— heartburn.

Of course there is no clear distinction between age groups; an infant can suffer from 'adult' problems and vice versa. They are listed this way for convenience, as some symptoms are more common in certain age groups.

Further, this is not a complete list, and it omits major disease. Among major chronic medical conditions sometimes linked with food intolerance are problems such as all forms of colitis, ulcers, vasculitis, seizures, respiratory arrest, phlebitis, cardiac arrhythmias, rheumatoid arthritis, other auto-immune diseases, renal disease including the nephrotic syndrome, postural proteinuria, membranous glomerulopathy, haemolytic anaemia, diabetes, schizophrenia.

One last point: parents are the 'experts' on their children. If you feel that one of your children 'just isn't right' for your family, whether in growth, health, or behaviour, check it our thoroughly. Doctors go on averages; they don't know you and your family situation in any detail. Hence they can easily put down to psychological causes what are in fact subclinical manifestations of intolerance or other disease. (And of course psychological factors are real, causing hormonal change and alterations in normal metabolism; they thus are potent triggers for intolerance problems.) Be completely honest with yourself in assessing this, though we all have our blind spots. If you feel that your child's behaviour is unreasonable in the context of how your family works, that given

101

his age, his parents' treatment of him, and the prevailing social factors, he ought to be better, then you are probably right in seeking further help. But it may take time to persuade anyone else of that!

The cumulative effect of small matters exerted over many years in human function is not generally appreciated. When erosion of a beach finally threatens the owner's cottage, he leaps into action. When the gradual attrition of disease produces obvious malfunction of a body part, the individual quickly seeks out a physician to effect a cure. He usually views the event, however, as one of recent origin, blissfully unaware of the years of accumulating small health deviations that have contributed to produce the acute event.

R. Wunderlich, *Allergy, brains and children coping.* J. Reads, Florida (1973).

11

What to do in pregnancy and lactation

The ideal time to sort out your food problems is before you become pregnant. New groups such as Foresight in the UK, and of course the NCT, are emphasizing the real benefits of preconceptual as well as prenatal care. If you are not pregnant but plan to have another child, and know yourself to have these problems, do take time to contact such groups. Even the time of year when your baby is born may be important in asthmatic families.[1] It is possible that within a few years local childbirth education groups may have incorporated this sort of information into their programmes.

However, what to do if you are now pregnant or breast-feeding. Unfortunately, in this crucial area there has been very little research. Many doctors are not willing to state publicly what they might privately agree with because the benefits of such routines are not scientifically proved, and therefore their colleagues might criticize, or patients blame them for less than perfect results.

Two suggested routines are given here. The first is adapted in part from patient advice sheets kindly provided by Professor R.N. Hamburger, Department of Pediatric Immunology and Allergy, University of California.

A. Maternal diet

1. Do not 'food binge' (eat any one food in excess) in pregnancy or while breast-feeding. Eat a balanced diet in moderation.
2. Avoid foods that you are allergic to, or which disagree with you. If pregnancy has made particular foods seem nauseating, avoid them.
3. Eat no whole eggs 1 month prior to birth, nor in the first months of breast-feeding. Limit your egg intake from all sources—cakes, mayonnaise, and so on.
4. Keep your intake of cows' milk below two glasses a day. (Drink none if you are sensitive to it.) Limit (or eliminate) other sources of cows' milk protien—cheese, ice cream, margarine, bread, and processed foods, etc. Add a calcium supplement if your intake is deficient.

103

Food for thought

5. Avoid as much as possible all food additives, artificial colourings and flavourings, preservatives, etc.
6. Limit or eliminate your intake of caffeine—coffee, tea, cola; also nicotine and alcohol. Take only prescribed drugs—and always ask whether the drug prescribed is safe in pregnancy or lactation. (It's easy for the doctor to forget that you are breast-feeding.) If vitamin or mineral supplementation is ordered, ask for hypo-allergenic formulations.
7. Do not go on elimination diets or experiment with discovering food sensitivities quickly.

B. Infant diet

1. Breast-feed your infant *exclusively* from birth, until at least 6 months or more. This may be the most important single preventive measure. See p. 188.
2. As a supplement or complement to breast-feeding in the rare instance where this is needed, use (a) your own frozen breast milk; (b) donated human milk; (c) amino acid, soy, or meat base formulae. Never give cows' milk formulae under at least 6 months.
3. If vitamin or mineral supplements are prescribed by a doctor, use *only* hypoallergenic ones. Disregard advice about orange juice or paediatric syrups. In general the exclusively breast-fed full-term infant requires no supplements. If you are concerned about your infant's vitamin status, improve your own. The breast readily excretes extra vitamin C and B, although it is very selective about what it does excrete into milk. Fluoride, for instance, is not excreted in large amounts even if mothers take large doses, although very similar chemicals are. Some researchers suggest that this may mean that the breast-fed infant is actively protected against large amounts of fluoride.
4. When introducing solid foods after 6 months be guided by the ideas in Ch. 15. (Since your child is less likely to be allergic if you have observed these guidelines, you have some leeway—use your common sense.)
5. Breast-feed for as long as you and baby enjoy it—remember that in many cultures children aren't weaned until 2–5 years old. Even a morning or night feed can only be valuable to the child, and it is extremely useful to be able to revert to full breast-feeding in episodes of illness. (Extra water is needed in the first days until supply builds up again, of course, or dehydration would be a risk.) I know of mothers feeding younger babies who have expressed milk for older children after gastroenteritis or bowel surgery. (One 3-year-old put on 500 g/day for a week on a mixed diet largely of human milk, egg, and soy.)

What to do in pregnancy and lactation

RECORD ALL ACCIDENTAL OR DELIBERATE VIOLA-
TIONS OF THESE RULES

C. General advice

1. Keep the house as free as possible of dust and moulds. Take special care with bedrooms—cf. Golos and Golbitz and Rapp in the Bibliography for details.
2. Ban all pets from the house for at least 6-months. (Cats are worse than dogs.)
3. Throw out as many chemicals as you can.
4. Don't smoke, or allow others to smoke near the baby, as far as is humanly possible, (see p. 52).
5. Don't subject your child to any *unnecessary* surgery or major stress in the first few years of life. This of course includes circumcision. It is not clear whether it is the pain, the anaesthesia, or some other factor, but it is quite clear that children who have had to undergo surgery have an abnormally high incidence of allergic disease.[2]

The University of California study, for which Professor Hamburger's guidelines were composed, was only a small one—some 50 mother–infant pairs. Patients were carefully matched with a control group, and all scientific precautions were taken. The results: 76 per cent of the study patients (cf. 36 per cent of controls) had experienced no major atopic disease by the age of two; more than twice as many study patients as controls had no atopic disease. (Data supplied by Professor Hamburger. This study has been expanded, and is continuing.[3]) Two points to note—I have adapted those original guidelines to include points found to be important by some mothers. Also, since we are concerned with 'minor' allergic disease, studies such as this simply do not go far enough. But the main point—that care with diet, etc., may help greatly in atopic families—emerges clearly enough, and was in fact confirmed by a careful UK study.[4] And if you stop and consider these guidelines, you'll realize that even if they do no real good, they should do no harm, at the very least. To be certain, discuss them with your doctor.

This second diet advice sheet was provided by Dr Del Stigler, a Denver paediatrician with special interest in this area. You will notice that there is a significant overlap between the two, and that both are compatible with the low-fat, low-salt, high-fibre diets now being almost universally recommended by health authorities.

Food for thought

Diet goals for pregnancy and nursing

1. Eat three meals per day: early morning, noon, and evening meal no later than 7:00 p.m., if possible.
2. A midmorning and midafternoon snack helps prevent nausea.
3. Meals and snacks should include a *protein* food (meat, raw seeds or raw nuts) and a *carbohydrate* (fruit, vegetables or grains).
4. Eat at least one raw fruit and one raw vegetable per day.
5. Drink 12 cups of liquid or more a day. Use only 100 per cent real fruit juices (no fruit drinks), spring water if possible, herbal teas (no maté in them), or plain, non-city water. (Boiling reduces chlorine content.)
6. Avoid coffee, black tea, decaffeinated coffee.
7. Eat all foods in as natural a form as possible, i.e. fresh and cooked, no processing, use whole grains.
8. Cook meats by wok, pan boil, flame broil, roast, or boil. Fry only twice monthly.
9. Eggs should be organic, from chickens that live on the ground, or from health food stores, if possible.
10. Use only cold processed oils (safflower, soy, sunflower seed, peanut). *Not* margarine. Butter may be used occasionally.
11. A craving for sweets may be satisfied with ripe, fresh fruit and/or larger portions of protein.
12. **Food choices**

Recommended foods		*Foods to avoid*
Grape-ade (carbonated mineral water with grape juice)	vs.	Pop (soft drink)
Raw nuts	vs.	Salted, dry roasted or oil roasted peanuts
Trail Mix (raw sunflower seeds with dried fruit)	vs.	Candy bar
2 fresh plums	vs.	Potato, corn, or cheese dips
Whole grain crackers	vs.	Soda crackers
Whole grain bread	vs.	Sweet roll
Rice cake with fruit puree	vs.	Doughnut

This topic is also discussed in Ruth Lawrence's book, *Breast feeding a guide for the medical profession,* pp. 345–6.

12

How to succeed at exclusive breast-feeding

The key to success is preparation—not of your body (nature takes care of that) but of your mind, and your relations! To succeed, it helps to have expert information, a supportive partner and/or family, and a good hospital.

What happens in the first week in hospital will determine how easily baby begins breast-feeding. For that reason it is worth shopping around, finding out beforehand what hospital policies and routines are like. No doctor or nurse nowadays would openly deny that 'breast is best', the evidence is overwhelming. However, it is one thing to say that the hospital encourages breast-feeding. It is quite another to have altered the routines that make failure likely, and to have persuaded nursing staff that formula is a desperate, even dangerous, last resort. Further it is rare to find experienced breast-feeding mothers among the nursing staff, and the management of the minor problems of lactation still leaves much to be desired. While I hope that you might find yourself in a really wonderful hospital with friendly, *skilled* and supportive staff, it is safer to work on the premise that you might not. So . . .

(A) IN PREGNANCY

1. Discuss with your doctor your desire to breast-feed, and ask for his support in the hospital situation. Discuss the advice given in earlier sections, and together periodically review your diet for nutritional adequacy. Ask your doctor to check your breasts. Should he discover an inverted nipple, it would be as well to consult the NCT's pamphlet on the subject.
2. Make contact with your nearest breast-feeding support group as early in pregnancy as possible. Begin to borrow books about breast-feeding, but most importantly, just be around at meetings where other mothers are feeding their babies. Soon it will seem like the most natural thing in the world. (For most of us it seems strange at first, because within our families we have not lived with breast-feeding.) The discussions you will be part of will give you a

Food for thought

far clearer idea of the realities of babyhood than any book—other than perhaps Penelope Leach's excellent volume, *Baby and child*.

3. Talk about all these things with your baby's father. His attitudes will be crucial to your success in feeding your baby. If he is aware of the advantages of breast-feeding and the real hazards of formula, he may be more willing to provide practical help after the birth, and important moral support in any conflict with hospital staff, family, and friends.

4. Talk about all these things with family and friends. Remember that the community in general has not been told of the hazards of anything but breast-feeding, and numerous old wives' tales circulate which can be very demoralizing if you hear them from a good friend on a day when your milk supply seems low. The more you educate your inner circle, the more help they will be to you afterwards. (And to other mothers too!)

5. If you intend to buy books, shop around. For my money the best—most detailed and reliable—book on breast-feeding is Helsing and Savage-King, although Stanway and Messenger both have much to recommend them. See bibliography for details. A book on child development—I like Leach's *Baby and child*—is also essential, though these are usually poor on breast-feeding matters. A selection of NCT pamphlets should also be packed in your hospital suitcase, along with this book.

6. If you have a freezer, stock up on simple ready-to-eat meals for the first months after baby's birth. Get in a supply of small boilable plastic or glass containers (ca. 4 oz) which can be used to store and freeze any excess milk expressed. If you can afford it, buy a hand-expressing and feeding bottle—or arrange to borrow one. Contact NCT about this, and buy their leaflet, *How to express and store breast milk*. Addresses for such bags and bottles are to be found in the resources section (p. 199).

7. Simplify the house as far as possible—for example, put away things that collect dust. Get in some good books that you have been wanting to read, or any other pastime that can be done one-handed; after the first few weeks you will not spend all of every feed time gazing enraptured at your child, but will enjoy the chance to relax and let him suck contentedly away. Make sure you have one very comfortable chair for feeding in—arm rests at the right height, good back support, ideally a foot-rest too. A small table nearby to put your book and a drink on is also a good idea.

How to succeed at exclusive breast-feeding

(B) IN HOSPITAL

1. Do feed baby as soon after birth as possible. (His sucking reflex is strongest at that time, so he learns fastest. His sucking stimulates the release of oxytocin and prolactin, hastening the production of milk. The colostrum he receives has a protective and laxative effect—and high levels of jaundice are associated with delayed opening of the bowels.)

2. Do feed baby as often as he likes—*ad libitum*—from birth unless he is very sleepy, and needs to be woken for feeding. Follow his cues, not any arbitrary schedule, but do feed at *least* six times a day. (Short frequent feeds are easiest on the nipples and best for your milk supply.)

3. Do ask that should extra fluid be medically essential in the first few days, this be plain water, not formula of any kind, and that it be given by dropper or spoon, not bottle. This is vital if supply

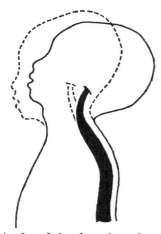

Angle of head and neck at which baby can feed and breathe easily.

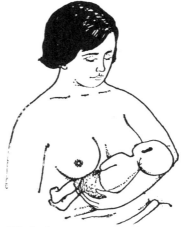

Mother's arm supports baby's head, but does not hold it in against the breast, rather, allows it to move at this angle. Chin touches breast when baby's body is close to mother's.

Fig. 12.1 Correct position of baby for breast-feeding. (From Gunther, M. (1970), *Infant feeding*, Methuen, London.)

109

and demand are to reach a state of balance. If you have any family history of allergy (asthma, eczema, hayfever, etc.) insist on this—until the gut lining has 'closed', baby is very likely to become sensitized to foreign protein, and so on. Bottle-feeding wrongly conditions a baby's sucking reflexes, and the ease with which milk flows may make him reluctant to work at the breast. Other fluids also seem to decrease weight gain,[1] and so cause staff to urge you to give complementary formula!

4. Do ask to night feed, at least after the first night. This is easiest if baby is 'rooming-in' but just as possible if he is not. See the night staff personally for best results. Feeding at night will keep any engorgement at reasonable levels.

5. Do take in some breast-feeding literature. You will be surprised how many new questions you and other mothers have. You need reliable answers immediately. Some hospitals stock such literature for mothers; most supply only women's magazines.

6. Do pay attention to correct position of the baby during feeds—mouth wide open against the areola, tongue well forward, lips turned out, chin against the breast, body close to yours, and lifted high enough so that he is not pulling on the nipple. The baby should be on his side, not on his back and turning his head sideways. And when he is well attached, if you gently press his bottom lip aside, you will see his tongue. If your nipples look flattened or feel sore after a feed, you're doing it wrong! For more detail consult Helsing and Savage-King's *Breast-feeding in practice,* or NCT's *Breastfeeding: Avoiding Some of the Problems.* Many nurses have not yet realized the logic of positioning and the ways in which this can be related to nipple problems and failure to thrive.

7. Do learn to recognize the 'let-down reflex' and never take the baby off the breast just as he is beginning to get his dinner—no matter what length of time you are being advised to feed for. (To restrict feeding times when the let-down is slow contributes to breast problems as well as leaving baby hungry.)

8. Do check your breast for lumpiness each night—especially towards the armpits and where the breast joins the chest wall. If you feel a lump, gently massage towards the nipple as baby feeds. Express if your breasts feel very overfull and painful. (This can always be given to other babies, or kept in case yours needs it later.) Remember this after you go home, especially when baby

sleeps longer than usual, or you have been wearing tight-fitting clothes.

9. Do experiment with finding comfortable feeding positions, both sitting and lying, while you have a nurse about to help you. Dont be afraid to take baby to bed with you and drowse off. If you are worried about baby falling out of such high narrow beds, put furniture/baby's trolley or somesuch up against the bed or take in a baby sling with extra long straps which can be loosely tied around both of you. Actually, babies snuggle up to warm bodies like homing pigeons, and your arm is quite enough protection—but hospital staff will be concerned about the hospital's liability. (Of course, you could always sign a form relieving them of responsibility.)

10. Do not take sleeping tablets or other optional drugs. They may make you clumsier with baby. They certainly disturb your normal sleep patterns; they may sedate the baby, so that she fails to suck vigorously; they lower the body's basal metabolism, decreasing milk production and of course, they don't help you to wake for night feeds, while they may also prove to be addictive in your case. That they are offered so freely to healthy people is nothing short of astonishing. I am told that 'normally rational and intelligent staff seem to suspend their brain function when it comes to handing out pills at night in UK hospitals.' True or false? If you have trouble sleeping in hospital, a set of ear plugs and an eye mask (such as provided by airlines) can be of help, along with your relaxation exercises.

11. Do be careful of your nipples. At the slightest sign of soreness, consult NCTs *Breastfeeding: avoiding some of the problems.* Remember, nothing drying or harsh should be used on nipples. If you have skin allergies, probably no cream is safest. If you try any, discontinue at the first sign of redness or soreness, and always test it first in some protected body crease such as the groin or elbow. If it causes redness over 24 hours, don't use it. The very latest advice is to express some hind milk and let it dry on the nipple. It provides natural body fats in their live form, complete with anti-viral, anti-bacterial, and anti-fungal properties. Don't scrub or soap up your nipples—normal showering is all that's required. If the hospital suggests using sterile swabs before and after feeds, remember that once you go home such tedious precautions are not necessary. Hospitals are dangerous places, with many disease-causing infectious agents that are not such a problem at home.

Food for thought

12. Don't be worried by 'test weighing' which is still routine in many hospitals. This sounds innocent enough, but it often means that mothers are not able to feed *ad libitum*, but must wait until sister is free to weigh the baby before and after. A 'top-up' twenty minutes later is usually frowned upon, and the very frequent little sucks that some babies like on some days are quite impossible.

Hospital staff *do* need to check that your baby is gaining weight, but this can be done quite satisfactorily without 'test' feeds, which create anxiety in the mother[2] and usually results in complementary feeding as staff decide that the baby could do with more than mother is supplying—on quite arbitrary and outdated calculations! One day of restricted schedule feedings, with anxiety over test results, is often enough to *cause* supply problems in mothers who were coping beautifully until then. So feel quite free to say no test weighs, thanks very much—unless of course your doctor insists, and explains why. Research published in 1981 actually indicates that testweighing is not always accurate.[3]

13. Don't believe that all nurses or doctors know much more about breast-feeding than you or the books you have. They are people too. Some nurses have never had a baby, some have bottle-fed theirs, some dislike the idea of breast-feeding (even if they can't say so as openly nowadays), some have arbitrary ideas as to which women are likely to succeed, some were taught almost nothing about breast-feeding, and so on. You will get very different advice from dozens of people and be thoroughly confused. Trust the experts, that is those women who have successfully breast-fed babies and enjoyed it, such as Dr Penny Stanway. But even then remember that you are unique, and so is your baby, and no rules can ever cover every situation. Trust yourself and your baby.

Do ring the nearest NCT counsellor or some other experienced breast-feeding mother or support person if you are having difficulties that seem insuperable. But remember, the more you express your feelings—and these will vary—the more likely it is that people will respond.

A basic hospital kit that has helped me:

- Eye mask—as given away in aeroplanes.
- Ear plugs—whatever sort are comfortable—helps with sleep in a noisy bright environment.

112

How to succeed at exclusive breast-feeding

● Your own pillow—well labelled, or with distinctive pillow-slips.

● An adapted baby sling with very long straps—to enable you to sleep safely with baby in bed beside you or to take her for walks.

● Small bottle of something alcoholic if alcohol helps you relax when tense. Definitely not to be overdone, as it decreases milk production and affects baby, but a mouthful just before feeds may help a delayed let-down. (This is a choice between evils—tension or a social drug.)

● Bed socks—plastic-coated mattresses are awful for my circulation!

● A decent muesli and plenty of fruit, to help with the bowels—why does no-one warn the new mother of this postnatal hazard?

● Good books on breast-feeding, for reassurance amid the sea of conflicting ideas.

(C) THE FIRST WEEKS AT HOME

Do not try to catch up on housework and friends, or do anything more than you can easily cope with. Remember that establishing a good supply of milk may take time, and the baby is your first priority. Do not be afraid to seek advice about trivial things—anxiety can be easily allayed. If you have any of the minor difficulties of breast-feeding, remember:

(1) It all gets easier as you go along, provided you learn from each experience. Persist until you get adequate help or explanation.

(2) No-one in the world can provide better for your baby than you. The problems of formula feeding are far more serious—though rarely talked about. And for the child of an allergic family they can be even more serious.

If you feel totally immersed in new baby and just coping, do not get anxious over how long that will last. The best way out of some things is through. Get baby settled and well fed, and you can gradually emerge and take up other activities. Try to force the pace and you may have a miserable demanding baby on your

113

Food for thought

hands. Ajusting your expectations to what is reasonable for your baby leads not only to happier babies but also happier parents. Read Penelope Leach's *Baby and child* for more detailed information about infant development.

If you have any extra milk express and store it.

If we are really serious in our attempts to bring back breastfeeding, milk bottles should be banned from hospital nurseries.

Gueri *et al. Journal of Tropical Paediatrics* **23(6)**, 267

Given adequate instruction, emotional support, and favourable circumstances, 96% of new mothers can successfully breastfeed . . . The benefits of breastfeeding to the neonate and the mother are so numerous that [physicans] must strongly encourage the practice . . .

American Academy of Pediatrics, 1979.

13

What to do for the colicky breast-fed baby

1. First of all, try all the standard remedies. Is baby too hot, too cold, too tired, too bored, too cramped? It would be a waste of effort to embark on what follows and then discover she was crying because of scalding urine on a sore bottom, or irritating prickly heat. Work your way through the list in for example, Penelope Leach's *Baby and child*, or NMAA's *Why is my baby crying?*, or read Kirkland or Jones (see p. 222).

2. If nothing works, and the doctor, ruling out any possibility of more serious problems, has diagnosed colic, you should stop to consider how and when she cries. Is it almost exclusively in the evenings for a few hours, settling down for a reasonable stretch at night? If so, what is your milk supply like? Does baby gulp greedily away at morning feeds, perhaps spluttering a bit, or even coming off the breast to allow the flow to settle down a little? The possibility here—and I would stress that this is a working hypothesis, nothing more—is of a transient, benign, lactose-intolerance colic. It could be that baby receives so much milk (with its high-lactose content) all at once in his small stomach that some of it is pushed through the intestines and not properly digested—there just is not enough lac*tase* to break it down when it all floods in. Consequently, by the evening—or roughly 12 hours after such a feed —the excess lactose has fermented causing gas, cramps (the colic) and general spasmodic pain. If this is the underlying mechanism, this colic could be prevented by:

    (a) increasing the size of baby's stomach, or the absolute amount of lactase in his gut—only time can do that! Has anyone looked to see whether growing out of colic corresponds to physical growth of stomach size, etc? Do small, slow-gaining babies take longer than big babies? Or is it enzyme levels in the gut that are critical?

    (b) Decreasing the amount of lactose which goes into that small stomach ALL AT ONCE. And many mothers have reported success by doing just that. Some practical ways are:

Food for thought

(i) To express before the morning feed, reducing the initial rapid flow. (Save the milk for the evening if need be, or freeze it for later use.) A Kaneson or other cylinder-type pump is useful for this.

(ii) To give a small quantity of plain boiled water before morning feeds, so that baby, feeling full sooner, switches off before having too much. (Of course he will need another feed sooner than before, but smaller, more frequent feeds have been demonstrated to be better for babies with lactose-intolerance diarrhoea.)[1]

(iii) To posture feed, or feed so that gravity is not assisting the flow of milk. See NCT's *Too much milk* for details.

(iv) To feed from only one breast at a time, which seems to reduce overall stimulation somewhat, and hence can only be recommended for those who know they have a plentiful supply overall. If baby receives only one breast, it usually takes him longer to feel full, so his non-nutritive suckling needs are met without making him over-full.

Babies with such a transient lactose-intolerance colic could be expected to be having fairly loose stools, but to be gaining weight well, as overall they are getting plenty of food. However, this is always a balancing act: if the lactose intolerance becomes too severe, damaging gut lining and causing the loss of more enzymes, including lactase, the baby could gain poorly or be at risk. So if loose stools become too frequent, the doctor's advice should be sought. Bear in mind the advice in Chapter 16 on the home management of diarrhoea, and the enormous variability of normal stools in a healthy breast-fed baby.

3. If that obviously is not your problem, and your baby just cries in a completely erratic fashion, consider the possibility of general food-intolerance colic. If the baby is still exclusively breast-fed, the problem must lie with something in your diet. Now here you have to be very sensible. A lactating mother cannot afford, for her own sake, to go in for drastic dietary changes, and abrupt changes in infant diet may do more harm than good. So begin to analyse the problem carefully. Read pp. 99–100—does that sound like you or your husband on a number of points? If so read Ch. 17. Begin by keeping a diet diary. List exactly what you have eaten for the last

What to do for the colicky baby

few days and pick out likely suspects. If you decide to eliminate one, or two, do it thoroughly and for at least two weeks—some babies take that long to settle down. If you decide to try challenges, remember that baby may react more sensitively than you—it can be a good idea to have milk expressed and frozen—with dates labelled—so that you can refer to your diet diary and see whether that day's milk is likely to produce colic or other symptoms. The breast-fed baby is a real aid to diagnosis of a mother's sensitivities. (Professor Matsamura and others are sure that if the child reacts, the mother has a problem too—even if she is not aware of it, having grown used to her symptoms. I'm not sure about that as yet.)

If baby is receiving solids or other fluids, including medications already, a period of exclusive breast-feeding may indicate whether the problem is in his diet or his mother's. However, watch that he receives enough fluid to avoid dehydration.

4. If none of the above helps, I would go back to the doctor for a very careful check-up. Baby may have overlooked physical problems such as gastro-oesophageal reflux—the acid from the stomach is causing pain. If your contented baby suddenly begins to scream in pain, don't just think 'colic'. It could be intestinal obstruction, which is potentially lethal unless corrected.

5. Keep fixed in your mind that babies don't cry like this for fun, to get attention, or to drive you crazy. If she sounds as though she is in pain, she probably is; so she needs your comfort in any form that helps. Baby slings can be a lifesaver. So can a recliner rocker, and a large family bed. (My basic parenting kit—scrimp on other things to acquire them.) Do not believe those who say you are spoiling her, that she will be all right if you just let her scream herself to sleep. How would you feel in a totally foreign country where you couldn't communicate your needs, and everyone ignored your distress? What sort of trust in life could develop from such isolated suffering? If you feel pushed to distraction by the lack of sleep—which is, after all, a form of torture around the world—get help wherever you can. We parents can't afford to be proud. She needs you, but she needs you sane. So do not take happy pills when under this sort of pressure—there is evidence that they may make you more prone to bursts of irrational rage, in which you might hurt baby. If you must, give her some mildly sedating anti-

Food for thought

histamine prescribed by your doctor—it could even help relieve her colic (see p. 88).

I really hope that's some help to you. It has been to dozens of parents, but there's no way of knowing what proportion of colic is due to either type of intolerance. Again, because 'he'll grow out of it', and because 'most women cope for that few months', it simply has not been a priority area of medical research. It's the partly self-inflicted ills of wealthy middle age that grab the headlines and the research funds.

In this section on colic, I have deliberately neglected to give importance to cultural expectations, maternal inexperience and anxiety, and other environmental and cultural influences. Why? Firstly, because parents hear all too much of them from other sources. (For a really first-rate review of such ideas and more, read Sandy Jones's book, *Crying babies, sleepless nights*.) Secondly, because there is no real evidence to support such ideas, despite the devotion with which male physicians repeat them. Yes, there are studies that show an association between colic and these factors. But, as doctors say when they want to discredit an unacceptable idea, associations can be explained in many ways. For example, maternal anxiety is an appropriate response to the experience of living with a crying baby—but what physiological mechanism exists to explain the notion that anxiety *causes* colic? In my experience, babies are remarkably placid through all sorts of family rows, so long as they are warm and well fed; while they will infallibly disrupt the most harmonious scene if they have a pain. Maternal inexperience results in such things as allowing nurses to give bottle-feeds, which may irreparably alter the normal development of extremely complex physiological systems in the infant. Inexperience leads mothers to try whatever anyone suggests from early solids on. Yet many multiparous mothers also have colicky infants—and they can usually understand why, after thinking about their and baby's, diet! Dietary hypotheses are inherently more plausible than the idea that mothers somehow give their babies gut-ache by being inexperienced or tense. A high association with certain anaesthetic agents (cf. pp. 30–1) could also have a dietary component as well as a drug effect—mothers who have difficult deliveries are also more likely to be separated from their

What to do for the colicky baby

babies in the first few days, more likely to have difficulty establishing lactation and so on.

Finally, I have disregarded these explanations because they are not helpful. To be told that irremediable factors like inexperience or anxiety are causing the problem which is driving you insane does nothing for maternal self-esteem or mother–child relationships. Husbands commonly interpret such statements as meaning that everyone else manages all right, but that their wife is incompetent—and that creates further tensions. (Indeed, this is a significant factor in marital distress and breakdown.) Physiological causes however, though difficult to pinpoint, hold out hope of improvement, reassure the mother of her competence, and thus enable her to be more compassionate and enduring in the meantime. Given our present epidemic of child abuse, much of it triggered by infant crying, these would seem to me very cogent reasons for avoiding unscientific waffle about maternal and cultural factors in the aetiology of colic. Such commonly held beliefs merely serve to provide excuses for not performing thorough physical investigations, and their widespread acceptance has been one of the obstacles to acceptance of the idea that food intolerance is involved. It has also delayed diagnosis of other physical problems, from reflux to urinary tract infections.

A major advance in the care of the newborn has often followed the observation that an accepted method of treatment has killed or maimed babies. Preterm infants were starved, cooled or blinded with O_2 until there was evidence that such treatments were dangerous. The newest hazard for the newborn infant is unnecessary separation from his mother.

H.B. Valman, *British Medical Journal*, **280**, 474 (1979).

14

But I'm bottle-feeding—what can I do?

Until some overdue changes are made, many women will unnecessarily bottle-feed their babies. While that may seem deplorable to me, it is fact. Many mothers want to know which formula, of those available, is best, safest, and so on. The only possible answer to that is—no-one knows.

We do know certain things:

1. Undiluted cows' milk is *totally* unsuitable for human infants—although it is still used in Australia, and probably the UK.

2. Home-made 'formulae', milk, water, and sugar, for example, are also utterly unsuitable for anything but emergencies. Evaporated, condensed, and dry milks, cow and goat and soy are included here. Whole generations of babies grew up on these, but nutritionally they are inferior to modern formulae and would not meet the guidelines referred to earlier (p. 42).

3. Some modern formulae are better than others, or so it seems. Ask local hospitals or health visitors which seem to be associated with most rashes, constipation and/or diarrhoea. My own experience is not wide enough to generalize on this. However, a recent analysis of the fatty acid composition of some Australian infant formulae[1] stated that while none exactly matched breast milk on that score (which may be impossible) only two, Nan and S26, had modified protein as well as electrolyte levels lowered to that of breast milk. Since they are closer (in that sense) to human milk, these may be preferable. I say 'may' because at this stage no-one knows. I am told that these are no longer available and the rough UK equivalents are Osterfeed, SMA Gold Cap, Cow & Gate Premium. You should consult your doctor or health visitor, who can check this for you.

4. Soy formulae are no less likely to cause allergy problems if given to young babies, and questions about their nutritional adequacy

are still unanswered. (No-one knows how to assess this really.) However, it may be less of a social handicap to be allergic to soy than to milk.

5. Hypo-allergenic formulae such as Pregestimil and Nutramigen do seem to have some advantages for the food-intolerant baby. In one recent study of colicky bottle-fed infants on cows' milk formulae, only 18 per cent improved on soy milks, while 53 per cent improved on Pregestimil (available in the UK on prescription only) or Nutramigen.[2] But don't rush to the chemists—these are expensive, and available cheaply only on prescription, most taste awful, though some babies don't mind; they may or may not be nutritionally as good as the so-called humanized formulae (Nan, S26, etc.) In the absence of comprehensive long-term large-scale, closely monitored evaluation of *each* product, it is hard to know whether these formulae are really suitable for anything but short-term use under medical supervision. Each new product is to some degree an experiment

6. Perhaps up to 10 per cent of children tried on these so-called hypoallergenic formulae still become intolerant of them as well, according to one speaker at a recent medical seminar on cows' milk intolerance.[3] If given from birth, perhaps many more would be intolerant of them. This seems to be evident from the history of soy formulae.

Not very cheering, is it? Which is why you ought to be asking hard questions of the medical authorities like 'why aren't mothers told of the hazards of bottle-feeding? What product can you recommend? etc.' But to get back to practicalities, I don't feel at all competent to advise you about what formula and so on—I really think you have to put that responsibility on to your doctor. Keep going back and asking for more help if the baby does not improve. It is because we mothers 'cope'—despairing of getting any more useful information—that nothing gets done. At present you will be considered to have a low tolerance threshold, or be slightly neurotic—but if all of us women really keep telling them what it's like to be stuck with a crying, sickly, miserable baby they may put more effort into finding solutions.

I have tried to consider what I would have done if I had been bottle-feeding my baby when he was so colicky. (Of course I would

Food for thought

have begun with 'humanized milk'.) I suspect I would have tried
soy formula. But knowing what I do now, I would have insisted on
the long-term prescription of a hydrolysed casein formula such as
Nutramigen, and refused challenges of cows' milk until he was 3 or
4 years old. As he was my only child, I would have tried to relactate. It is quite possible to go back to breast-feeding even after
months and years. (But it is not something everyone can do or
would want to. See Avery's book, p. 214, and talk to an NCT
breast-feeding counsellor.) It would seem sensible, once the child
is past 4 months or so, to reduce the total quantity of any one
allergen by widening the diet, even though this carries the risk that
the child may become intolerant of other foods as well. Sometimes
these children cope with a mixed diet more easily than with exclusive milk feeding, even of the best formula. However, if the child is
totally milk-intolerant there are other alternatives. A World
Health Organisation Sub-Committee on Nutrition has formulated
detailed guidelines for the dietary management of young infants
who are not adequately breast-fed. This has been published in full
in Helsing and Savage-King, pp. 226–44, and is available from the
World Health Organization (see p. 202). Some of these gruels,
while time-consuming to prepare, might be more palatable and
nutritious than some of the expensive specialized formulae.
Perhaps allergy groups could invest in a copy of Helsing and
Savage-King for the group library? Talk about this option with a
nutritionist.

One thing to avoid is rapid formula changes, switching from one
to another and back again. If, on medical advice, you decide to
change, do so thoroughly and for at least 2 weeks. Experimenting
may result in multiple allergies—hence the need to discuss your
proposed course of action, and think it through before you begin.

Other than that, I cannot offer much help. I am really sorry if all
this information about the inadequacies of formulae is upsetting.
But somehow people must discover these things, so that informed
decisions can be made in future. Try to keep it all in perspective
(see p. 39). And help us work for the day when the State accepts
its responsibility to provide human milk for human babies who
need it. New York State has legislated to set up milk banks—if the
blood banks can solve the technical and ethical problems involved,
so could milk banks. That will be too late for you, I realize. Do
keep reassuring yourself that your baby's colic is not your doing

But I'm bottle-feeding—what can I do?

(see p. 118); that she may have been colicky when breast-fed. If you find other information that would help bottle-feeding mothers, please let me know—this is the only aspect of the book that I really dislike.

Most mothers who do not breastfeed are acting out of ignorance rather than intent . . . Education is mandatory at each step of the perinatal process

The influence of hospital staff in the decision to breast or bottle feed is stronger than we would like to believe . . . a decision regarding breast or bottle feeding isn't finalized until the baby is born . . . the hospital staff play a very important role in not only the woman's decision to breast or bottle feed, but also their ability to follow through their decision . . .
An administrative petition to alleviate domestic infant formula misuse
pp. 72, 70, Salisbury & Blackwell (1981).

123

15

How to introduce other foods to the potentially or actually intolerant baby

First of all, stop and think again, from first principles. No-one can tell you exactly what to do because no-one but you knows the degree of your sensitivity, what foods you ate in pregnancy, what minor symptoms your baby has manifested while fully breast-fed etc. What you do must be modified by what *only you* know.

Secondly, remember that for as long as your baby is gaining weight fairly consistently, and is obviously alert and healthy in other ways, there is no need to give extras, so you have time to think this all through first. Do not rush into it. Remember that the introduction of other foods actually decreases the bioavailability of nutrients in breast milk, and alters baby's gut bacteria.

Do not do it until you have to.[1] This will vary. Almost all women can breast-feed exclusively for 4–6 months; some can give the baby nothing else for 9–12 months. But it is not a competition. Once your baby is not gaining adequately on breast milk alone, he needs other foods. (I am assuming that a careful investigation of the 'how' of breast-feeding has taken place—slow gains in some breast-fed babies are the result of poor suckling technique.[2] And I am also assuming that such babies would be at least 4 months, as even malnourished mothers feed adequately for the first few months.)

Thirdly, remember the conflicting ideas outlined on pp. 21–3. Some state that you should vary the food, others urge that you keep the exposure small but constant. Decide what seems most reasonable to you and then give it a serious trial. If you suffer severely from food intolerance, a rotary diversified diet[3] may be the best idea, but involves a lot of work and reorganization— which would be beyond me!

If salicylate sensitivities are evident, omit or further delay the introduction of such foods (see *The Feingold cookbook*, Random House, 1979). This is not very common, however, as a *sole* source of problems.

Foods for the intolerant baby

If you have problems keeping up a sufficient supply of milk after four or five months, contact your local breast-feeding support group for help. If the baby needs more food than you can supply after following their suggestions, it may be necessary to vary these guidelines, although donated breast milk can help you through a temporary shortage. It is worth thinking ahead if you know yourself to be allergic and think baby could be at risk: in the early days many women express and freeze any excess milk (See NCTs *How to Express and Store Breast Milk*.)

If the problem is one of low supply in the evenings, try feeding baby on one side and simultaneously expressing the other breast into a Kaneson pump at the early morning feeds. Save the milk for evening, and let baby suck as long as he likes on the expressed breast. After a week you will be producing the extra volume in the morning and still have a few spare ounces for the evening hungry period. (Baby may still need to suckle during the evening, or the lack of stimulation might cause your supply to drop.) Mine all suffered 'six o'clock starvation', and stayed at the breast all evening, until I hit upon this idea and then Elizabeth slept 12 hours solid. (I expressed before going to bed so as to avoid engorgement over such a long period.)

But remember—should baby's weight gain be consistently poor, consult your doctor or clinic sister, and persist in seeking help. Some babies are meant to be small, of course—but if baby is born an average weight and both parents are average, persistent slow growth needs investigation. But don't judge the breast-fed infant by comparison with formula-fed babies—a heavier mineral load inevitably makes a bigger and heavier baby. That does not mean healthier.

The following suggestions reintroduction of foods are modified from a leaflet produced by the Allergy Information Association, Room 7, 25 Poynter Drive, Weston, Ontario M9R 1K8 Canada. Write for their list of information letters—very helpful yet inexpensive.

It is unfortunate that so far only parent self-help groups have attempted to provide such practical guidelines. Once again, the risk of being seen to do something 'not scientifically proven' seems to make professionals reluctant to tackle the harder issues. So this guide can only be provisional, and based on the experience of

Food for thought

Table 15.1 Introducing solid foods to the allergic baby

1. Avoid being sensitized by the most common foods to cause allergies, e.g. milk, wheat, eggs, corn, tomatoes, citrus, by leaving them as late as possible to the diet.
2. Introduce foods one at a time in order to avoid confusion should there be an allergic reaction.
3. To introduce a food, give the baby only a teaspoon on the first day. On the second day give the baby two teaspoons. Go on adding another teaspoon each day until the baby has a complete serving. If you suspect that the child may be sensitized to the food, go more slowly. If the baby rejects any food, do not persist in offering it, or disguise its taste. Babies are often aware of the limits of their own tolerance of foods. To overcome that rejection may lead to 'addiction'.
4. While introducing a food, watch very carefully for allergic symptoms, such as those on p. 33.
5. If none of the symptoms show up during the introduction to the food, then it can be considered a safe food, although it should not be eaten too often or too much at once.
6. If one or more of the symptoms appear, then stop the food, wait a week, begin a new food.
7. Keep a written record of the food, amount, symptom, or lack of symptoms.
8. When not testing a food, avoid giving the same food in a run. Vary the foods as much as possible.

Vitamins
If prescribed, use hypoallergenic only, that is free of lactose, yeast, wheat, etc. There is usually no need for *any* vitamin supplementation in Australia while the child is *fully* breast-fed; certainly not under 6 months. Introduction of other foods alters absorption of certain nutrients in breast milk, especially minerals such as iron. The best way to supplement a breast-fed baby is to supplement his mother's diet—the levels in milk are affected by diet.

Cereal
Six months, single grain variety, not mixed cereal. Begin with oatmeal, barley, or rice. Leave wheat until 9 months.

Fruit
At 5–6 months. First try pears, apricots, and prunes. Then mashed bananas (ripe). Leave apples and peaches until 12 months. Leave raw fruit until 12 months. Leave citrus fruit until 18 months. Leave berries until 24 months.

Milk
Nurse baby as long as possible, ideally, until the baby is at least a year. Nurse *ad libitum*; never try to force a schedule on to the baby. He will create his own. Introduce dilute juices in a cup at about 6–9 months.

Foods for the intolerant baby

If baby appears to be allergic to breast milk, it could be foods the mother is eating. She should avoid the common allergy foods, then test. If a supplementary milk is needed after 5 or 6 months exclusive breast-feeding, either cows' milk or soy formulae can be tried. If giving extra fluid because of temporary low supply and very hot weather, give either plain boiled water (under 6 months) or diluted formula. Only when it is baby's *sole* or *major* source of nourishment must you adhere rigidly to the directions for making up a milk formula or risk malnutrition. Remember that babies may be able to tolerate a certain amount of formula, but too much on one day or over a few days may overcome their tolerance. Watch baby's weight gain for indicators. However, a hungry baby may become lethargic, so make sure he gets plenty to eat overall (breast milk, formula, and other foods).

Vegetables
At 4–6 months. First try carrots, pumpkin, marrow, sweet potatoes, cabbage, cauliflower, broccoli, turnips, white potatoes. Leave beans, spinach, and peas until one year. Leave tomatoes until $1\frac{1}{2}$ years. Leave corn until 2 years.

Eggs
Leave until 12 months. Start by giving a quarter of a teaspoon of yolk only of a hard boiled egg, three times a week at most. Then increase by half a teaspoon at a time, until baby can eat the whole yolk without symptoms. Once he is used to the yolk, give him very small amounts of egg white, only gradually increasing it.

Meat
At 6–9 months. Try lamb, veal then beef, then pork–leave liver and chicken to the last, unless the chicken is free range fed. Watch veal and beef if the child is milk intolerant—both contain some of the same proteins as milk.

Fish
Leave until 12 months—start with a non-oily white-fleshed fish.

Chocolates and nuts
Leave until 2–3 years at least. Nuts are dangerous for the child under 5, who may easily inhale them. If they are given, it should be under close supervision, one at a time and well chewed, unless of course they are ground up.

If you feel that you are tempted to go faster than this schedule, remember: The baby doesn't need it. It is you that 'needs' variety.
Fast feeding is beneficial to the baby food companies, not your baby.
Fast feeding is a symptom of our hurry, hurry world. Until the 1920s few mothers fed solids to their children under a year old. Above all, remember that how you feed the baby in his first year may affect him all his life. He will be what he eats.

Food for thought

Canadian parents and doctors. I sincerely hope that some other groups will be spurred to tackle this question.

If your baby has shown no real signs of allergy, there is no need to be overly concerned about how to introduce solids. Good general guides are Salter, Helsing and Savage-King, Messenger, and NCTs *Introducing solid food.* (See Bibliography.)

WHAT IS A HEALTHY DIET FOR A YOUNG CHILD?

Here in Australia, we hear a lot about high-fibre, low-fat, low-carbohydrate diets where many of us could afford to lose weight (*Mea culpa!*) In their concern to do the best thing for their children, some parents have gone to extremes. Children's needs are different, because they are actively growing. They have only small stomachs, and high-fibre diets may fill them up without providing the calories they truly need. While this malnutrition is common around the world where protein and fats are in short supply, doctors tell me they are seeing it here as parents refuse to give their children animal products, fats or oils, or any nutrient-dense foods. So remember, a diet that suits an adult may not be adequate for a child. Consult a dietitian; many more are working in the community these days. Let the dietitian assess your child's diet, and then be guided by the dietitian's recommendations. Just as a constant diet of hamburgers, milk-shakes and chips would cause problems for a child, so would a diet of low-calorie, high-fibre foods. (Protein —calorie malnutrition, it's called in the textbooks).

WHAT ABOUT CALCIUM?

Children and, perhaps even more, their mothers need an adequate daily intake of calcium. This need not come from milk products, of course. The milk-intolerant person is quite likely not to absorb many nutrients in milk if the symptoms include gut reactions, and no one wants strong bones at the expense of good health. Milk is emphasized so much in Australia partly because it *is* a good source of available calcium, but largely because it is an economically important product. If there were more soybean producers, we might hear about the value of bean curd as a source of protein, calcium, and other minerals. But what do we use when milk is off the menu?

128

Table 13.2 Calcium supplements

	Amount of elemental calcium per dose	Wholesale cost per dose	Cost per 500 mg elemental calcium	Cost per day's therapy
Sandocal 1000 Effervescent tablets $4.00/30 (NHS) (authority required) $7.33 (over the counter)	1000 mg	24.4c/tablet 13.3c/tablet[a]	12.2c 6.65c[a]	$\frac{1}{2}$ tablet/day = 500 mg Ca = 12.2c 6.65c[a]
Spar-Cal Effervescent tablets $4.00/100 (NHS) (authority required) $12.33 (over the counter)	500 mg	12.3c/tablet 4c/tablet[a]	12.3c 4c[a]	1 tablet/day = 500 mg Ca = 12.3c 4c[a]
Calcium gluconate 600 mg tablets $2.76/100	53.5 mg	2.76c/tablet	25.8c	10 tablets/day = 535 mg Ca = 25.8c
Calcium lactate 300 mg tablets $2.21/100	38.9 mg	2.21c/tablet	28.4c	12 tablets/day = 467 mg Ca = 28.4c
Calvita tablets 450 mg calcium phosphate $3.43/100	174.4 mg	3.43c/tablet	9.83c	3 tablets/day = 523 mg Ca = 9.83c
Calcium powder (Hamilton's) citrus flavoured 4 g = 1300 mg Calcium gluconate $9.16/375 g powder $4.55/125 g powder also	116 mg/4 g	9.77c/4 g dose	42.1	4 × 4 g/day = 464 mg Ca = 42.1c

[a]Cost to the patient if obtained as a Pharmaceutical Benefit.   Note: Costs based on approximate retail price at January 1984.

129

Food for thought

Various calcium supplements exist, and many parents rely on these alone. Some assume that a 500 mg tablet of calcium gluconate provides the recommended daily allowance (RDA) for children, which is 400–800 mg. Alas, less than 10 per cent of the tablet is calcium; you would need to give the child 10 tablets daily at a ridiculous cost. It is inexcusable that such products are sold without any indication of their true calcium content or the amount needed to meet the RDA, when even breakfast cereals tell us that much. In a recent article in the *Journal of Food and Nutrution*, Melbourne dietitians published details of such supplements, which I am reproducing with their permission.

Perhaps some UK dietitians could produce a similar table for local products. While the costs are not relevant, the small quantities of calcium available from quite large tablets holds good.

Other supplements available include dolomite powder (calcium and magnesium, mainly), which is cheap to buy but is not well absorbed, and bone powder (calcium, phosphorus, and other minerals as found in ox bones). Both these products are tasteless and largely additive-free; they can be added to soups, stews, and home-made biscuits and bread. Ask your dietitian for further information and for an assessment of our family's diet. Perhaps you are getting enough protein, calcium, and other minerals into your children by your particular combination of foods. (Although this difficult when milk is entirely omitted from an average diet, your diet may not be 'average'.)

The increased number of children with allergies is ample evidence that there may be a relationship between early infant feeding methods and the subsequent development of intolerance to different substances. The fact that as many as 10% of all artificially fed babies are allergic to cows' milk should also act as a signal that there may be a more efficient way to feed infants, one that is less likely to cause such early and profound feeding difficulties, one that is less emotionally and financially expensive, and one that is easier on the child's digestive system.

K.G. Auerbach, in *Keeping Abreast Journal*, July–Sept (1976).

16

Home management of diarrhoeal disease

The need for this section of the book has become very obvious over the last few years of following up intolerant families. Diarrhoea is said to affect 10–40 per cent of all Western infants in the first year of life. (It kills around 18 million children annually.) Diarrhoea and vomiting can be caused by bacteria, viruses, and food/inhalants, among other things. The intolerant person is more readily affected by all three. Among food-intolerant families diarrhoea and vomiting can be responsible for long-term malabsorption, failure to thrive, and minimal brain deficits. Unfortunately community education about diarrhoea has been almost non-existent in the Western world. It is the basis of remarkably successful programmes in the developing countries which are finally, in December 1982, being noticed by the Western press.

The Director-General of UNICEF, Mr James Grant, was quoted as saying, 'The need for oral rehydration therapy (ORT) is clear, the technology is known, the means of dissemination are available. The receptiveness of parents has been demonstrated. The cost is small. And only an inexcusable lack of national and international will can now prevent the bringing of its benefits to the vast majority of children in need.'[1]

There are those who would dispute that Western children fit that category of 'need' because we have a relative oversupply of doctors. Personally I agree with Dr Jelliffe that ORT has 'more relevance to maternal and child health, particularly among disadvantaged and underserved groups, in industrialized countries than is often appreciated.[2] Any child can become dehydrated and suffer brain damage or die whatever its parent's income. Simple reluctance 'to be a nuisance', or the wish not to be thought 'overanxious' can delay by hours the beginning of appropriate treatment. We may have a lot of doctors, but many are not readily available nowadays. The number of children admitted to hospital for intravenous rehydration should be seen as an indictment of the failure of community health education. It is my hope that authorities in every developed nation will formulate a simple pro-

131

tocol for the home management of diarrhoea, and publicize it widely. It may be that this WHO recipe, designed for Third World conditions, should be altered for Britain. However, so long as additional free water is offered, and all the instructions followed, there is a considerable safety margin. The use of specifically designed measuring spoons also increases the safety of home management, so write to TALC today (see p. 197) and get a set for your bathroom cupboard. Alternatively, go out to the chemist and buy some Dioralyte or Dextrolyte. It should keep indefinitely. Remember to consult your doctor and do not accept lengthy waiting for appointments. Children can dehydrate and die in a matter of hours.

This guide to prevention and treatment has been adapted, with permission, from a leaflet produced by AHRTAG (Appropriate Health Resources and Technology Action Group), 85 Marylebone High St., London WIM 3DE. The measurements given have been checked by an anonymous research nutritionist and friend. My thanks to her and to AHRTAG (a group with many of the world's experts in this subject on its Board and funded by the UN Development Project, etc.)

I have put the guide in here, complete, despite some repetition because in dealing with diarrhoea parents need all the information to hand. This is not intended to discourage parents from consulting their doctor. He alone can do the tests needed to discover whether the diarrhoea is bacterial in origin and whether antibiotics are thus needed. (It is usually viral, or food-induced.) Once he rules out that possibility, the major risk is that of dehydration. Ask his opinion of this guide and **let him know that you are using it.**

The following guide includes:

1. Diarrhoea and dehydration
2. Assessing the severity of a patient's condition
3. Management
   - Treatment plan A: diarrhoea without dehydration
   - Treatment plan B: diarrhoea with mild dehydration—preparing and giving Oral Rehydration Salts Solution.
   - Treatment plan C: diarrhoea with severe dehydration—Going to hospital and what to expect.
4. Prevention.

Home management of diarrhoeal disease

1. DIARRHOEA AND DEHYDRATION

(1) The danger of diarrhoea is the body's loss of WATER and SALTS, that is DEHYDRATION.

(2) Dehydration can be prevented by giving more breast milk, water, and other drinks than normal **as soon as diarrhoea starts**.

(3) Dehydration can be treated by giving oral rehydration salts (ORS) solution **as soon as the dehydration starts**, or as soon as possible thereafter.

(4) Oral rehydration salts solution can be made by anyone at home provided extreme care is taken not to vary the recipe from that given. Commercial ORS mixtures are available from any chemist, together with instructions in their use. You should have a packet in your medicine cupboard.

(5) Where possible, follow this plan of action in conjunction with your local doctor, who can rule out other possible serious causes of diarrhoea. However, begin treatment immediately—do not wait until after seeing the doctor.

2. HOW SEVERE IS THE PATIENT'S CONDITION?

Table 16.1 Assessing the severity of diarrhoeal disease

1. **ASK**	DIARRHOEA	Less than 4 liquid stools per day	4–10 liquid stools per day	More than 10 liquid stools per day or much blood and mucus
	VOMITING	None or small amount	Some	Very frequent
	THIRST	Normal	More than normal	Unable to drink
	URINE	Normal	Small amount, dark	No urine for 6 hrs.
2. **LOOK**	CONDITION	Well, alert	Unwell, sleepy or irritable	Very sleepy, floppy, unconscious having fits or seizure
	EYES	Normal	Sunken	Very dry and sunken
	MOUTH and TONGUE	Wet	Dry	Very dry
	BREATHING	Normal	Faster than normal	Very fast and deep

133

Food for thought

Table 16.1 (*Cont.*)

3. **FEEL** SKIN	Pinch goes back quickly	Pinch goes back slowly	Pinch goes back very slowly
PULSE	Normal	Faster than normal	Very fast, weak or cannot be felt
FONTANELLE (in infants)	Normal	Sunken	Very sunken
4. **WEIGH** if possible (1 gram of weight gain/loss = 1 gram of fluid retained/lost)	No weight loss during diarrhoeal illness	Weight loss of 25–100 g for each kg of of weight	Weight loss of mo⟩ than 100 g for eac⟩ kg of weight
5. **TAKE TEMPERATURE** if possible	—	—	High fever 102°F 39 °C
6. **DECIDE**	If the child or adult with diarrhoea is like this there is NO DEHYDRA-TION	Ithe child or adult with diarrhoea has *2 or more of these signs* there is DEHYDRA-TION	If the child or adul with diarrhoea has 2 or more of these DANGER SIGNS there is SEVERE DEHYDRATION
	USE PLAN A	USE PLAN B	USE PLAN C

3. HOW TO MANAGE DIARRHOEA

The following treatment plans are written for young children but they can be used for **all** patients. For older children and adults exactly the same steps should be followed (except those about infant feeding); where the treatment plan says 'child' or 'mother' put in the word 'patient'.

In older children and adults, **thirst** is the best guide to treatment of dehydration. They should drink as much ORS solution as they wish. **Plain water** *and* **other fluids** should also be available for them to drink whenever they wish. They should start to eat a normal diet as soon as they are hungry: they should not wait until the diarrhoea stops.

Treatment plan A: diarrhoea without dehydration

1. **Continue feeding the child:**

— Breast milk as often as he wishes to suck, or can be

134

Home management of diarrhoeal disease

persuaded to; or in any other way—spoon, dropper, bottle . . .;

— other clear liquids (e.g. diluted juices, very weak teas, boiled water, rice water, etc.) in more than usual amounts.

— if the child is bottle-fed, any formula he receives should be mixed with an equal volume of water until the diarrhoea stops.

— if the child is already receiving solid foods, he may continue to eat small quantities of easily digestible foods as often as he wishes. However, avoid giving him too much of any one food at a time, and avoid foods that have caused him any reactions in the past, as well as very sweet, very salty, or very rich foods. (A breast-feeding mother should also avoid these and any known allergens—hers or the baby's.)

2. **Weigh the child and record the weight** (where possible)
In a very young baby this is especially important. Daily weight is a good indicator of fluid balance, as every gram of weight gained or lost indicates a gram of fluid retained or lost. See Table 16.1.

3. **Watch for the signs of dehydration:** (see Table 16.1)

— little or no urine; darker colour and stong smell;
— fast, weak pulse;
— sunken, tearless eyes:
— dry mouth (lips, tongue, gums);
— sunken fontanelle in babies;
— loss of normal skin elasticity or stretchiness—a pinch of skin goes back into place only slowly;
— lethargy, sleepiness.

If these signs develop, proceed to treatment plan B or C as appropriate (see Table 16.1). If in any doubt obtain medical advice immediately.

Treatment Plan B: Diarrhoea with mild dehydration

When some dehydration has occurred, ORS solution will be needed to replace the salts and water lost. *Other extra fluids should continue to be given, as in treatment plan A.* Above all, the mother should continue to breast-feed as frequently as before, and to be careful of her own diet, with particular attention to avoiding her

Food for thought

own known allergens and all unnecessary drugs, including tea, coffee, and cigarettes.

1. Preparing home-made ORS solution

(a) Go to the cupboard and make up the commercial ORS solution *exactly* as is stated on the box or the leaflet in it. Read all the instructions carefully. These solutions are quite different from the WHO formula, but many doctors consider commercial products safer than home made.

(b) If you have no commercial mix, you can make your own. The basic ingredients are salt and sugar. The underlying principle is that in certain concentrations, salt, sugar, and water are well absorbed, but in weaker or stronger concentrations they are not (and indeed, may actually cause further fluid loss). So it is really important to get the quantities right. The varying size of a teaspoon makes this difficult. However, special measuring sets are available, (see p. 132). But in an emergency, a teaspoon will have to do. (You can check whether it is standard 5 ml size by using a dropper to put 5 ml of water on to it and noting the level.) If in doubt, use your smallest teaspoon, not your largest. To a jug of a litre of cool boiled water add:

FUNDAMENTAL INGREDIENTS

(1) 1 flat teaspoon of cooking salt
(2) 4 flat teaspoons of *Glucodin
     Glucodin (dextrose) is used rather than ordinary white sugar (sucrose) because sucrose is a problem for many food-intolerant children; and because Glucodin contains small amounts of vitamin B6. However, sucrose *can* be used; it requires twice as much sucrose (i.e. 4 heaped teaspoons) to supply the same amount of usable glucose. If there is no Glucodin in the pantry, it is better to use white sugar than to wait until powdered glucose (dextrose) can be bought.

If you have them on hand, you can also add:

(3) ½ flat teaspoon of potassium bicarbonate (available from any chemist)
     Potassium bicarbonate in these quantities replaces the potassium lost in the stools. However, other dietary sources of potas-

136

Home management of diarrhoeal disease

sium are oranges and bananas. If you cannot quickly obtain potassium bicarbonate, offer your child these in some form until you can do so.

(4) 1/10th flat teaspoon of sodium bicarbonate (**absolutely no more**)

IT IS ALWAYS SAFER TO UNDERESTIMATE THESE INGREDIENTS THAN TO OVERESTIMATE THEM.

Be scrupulous in measuring them, and begin with a little **more** than a litre of boiled water so as to give you more of a margin for error (since teaspoons vary considerably in size.)

NEVER decide that 'about this much looks OK' Too much bicarbonate for instance can fatally disturb the body's acid/base balance. None is safer than too much.

2. Giving ORS solution

(A) How much to give?

THESE ARE GUIDELINES ONLY. IF THE PATIENT WANTS MORE ORS SOLUTION, GIVE MORE. IF THE EYELIDS BECOME PUFFY, STOP GIVING THE SOLUTION AND CONTINUE GIVING OTHER LIQUIDS. START ORS SOLUTION AGAIN WHEN PUFFINESS IS GONE AND IF DIARRHOEA CONTINUES. ALLOW FREE ACCESS TO PLAIN BOILED WATER AS WELL AS OTHER SUITABLE FLUIDS. (SEE TREATMENT PLAN A.)

Table 16.2 How much ORS to give   (all measurements in ml)

Child's weight in kilograms (1kg=2.2lbs)		3 4	5 6 7 8	9 10 11	12 13 14	15 20 30 40 50
For the first 4–6 hrs of dehydration give: (see Treatment Plan B)		200 400	400–600	600–800	800–1000	1200 2500 4500 1500 3500
For continual diarrhoea and to prevent dehydration from coming back use Method 1 or 2	M1—After every diarrhoea stool give:	50	100		150	200 300 350 400
	M2—Over 24 hrs give:	400	600	800	1000	2500

137

Food for thought

(B) How to give ORS solution
(i) By any means acceptable to the child—cup, spoon, bottle, eye-dropper, or nursing supplementer.
(ii) In small amounts. If the child vomits, wait 5 minutes or so and then give more. (Some is retained.) Continue to do so.
(iii) Keep the child under close observation. If his condition worsens, go direct to hospital. If he refuses to drink, go direct to hospital.

(C) After 4–6 hours of this treatment, check the child for signs of dehydration
If the child is taking ORS solution well but some signs of dehydration remain, give the same amount again in the next 4–6 hours. If the infant is breast-fed, continue to offer the breast freely. Remember that the baby may be able to cope well with small frequent feeds but not with large 3 hourly ones, as he may become temporarily lactase-deficient (cf. pp. 7–9).

If the infant is not breast-fed give 100–200 ml of plain boiled water before continuing the ORS solution.

Repeat this procedure until the signs of dehydration have gone, unless the child is clearly becoming worse. You must observe him closely over this period. If in any doubt, go to hospital.

(D) After the signs of dehydration have gone
If the child is still having diarrhoea, look at Table 16.2 and see how much ORS solution he needs for maintenance to prevent signs of dehydration developing. Give this amount until the child's stools have returned to normal. In addition, start feeding the child and continue giving other fluids as in treatment plan A. Feed him frequently until stools are normal, and continue to offer extra food for a week or more, so that the child can make up his losses. Once again, however, be sensitive to the possibility that some foods may cause relapses if the child is intolerant of them. Never coax or coerce a child to eat food that he dislikes, or more of it than he wishes at one time. Offer him a widely varied selection of foods, without too great a dependence on the most common allergens (milk, wheat, egg, etc.)

Treatment plan C: severe dehydration

1. If the child can drink, start ORS solution or any other suitable fluid as in plan B while waiting for transport and on the way to the

nearest hospital. Call a taxi or ambulance if you have no car and can afford to do so, or ask a friend to drive you there.

2. If visiting a doctor, emphasize to the receptionist that this is a seriously ill child and waiting is simply not advisable. If your local doctor is not available, go directly to hospital and call him later.

3. When at the hospital, INSIST on having your child seen to promptly. Once the danger signs are present, the child is at risk of brain damage or death. Continue to breast-feed frequently and give ORS solution while waiting.

4. Once your child is admitted and doctors have advised you of the proposed plan of treatment, do all you can to co-operate with the staff while remaining with the child. It is sometimes necessary for breast-feeding to be briefly interrupted if the child is losing weight rapidly and is seriously lactose-intolerant. (This is a clinical judgment, based *not only* on the result of the simple test for lactose but also on the volume, frequency, and character of his stools, and his general condition.) When the child is seriously ill, mothers should accept such a brief interruption gracefully—it should be a matter of days, not weeks, and the mother can express her milk. In some hospitals this will be diluted with water and fed to her baby. However, if the decision to stop breast-feeding seems almost automatic, and is based *solely* on the test for lactose, the mother should be aware that there are other schools of thought. She is within her rights to ask for an explanation or to seek a second opinion. It is usually fairly clear whether the hospital staff appreciate the unique protective and nutritional value of human milk, and do all they can to support breast-feeding mothers. If it is not clear to you, ask the doctors what their policy is about breast-feeding and gastroenteritis. If it becomes clear that the staff consider cessation of breast-feeding a trivial matter, and see no problems in the use of lactose-free formulae, the mother is entitled to ask them to consider the latest research findings, and to continue breast-feeding meanwhile, particularly if she suspects her child to be food-intolerant. A sudden switch from human milk to substitutes can cause serious problems. However, mothers should do their best not to antagonize staff by any signs of mistrust or opposition. It would be a pity if this resulted in mothers being 'difficult' for staff who are as reluctant as they are to see a baby off the breast. The

Food for thought

issue has been raised simply because there are, regrettably, a few doctors and nurses who are unware of the latest breast-feeding research and are unduly trusting of 'scientific' formulae, despite all the problems of such foods.

5. The child with severe dehydration may or may not require intravenous rehydration, that is he may be put on 'a drip'. This does not prevent continued breast-feeding, or oral fluids as well. If your baby wishes to breast-feed, a little boiled water before feeding will effectively dilute your milk. However, some experts consider even this unnecessary because with frequent suckling human milk tends to become more dilute in any case. When mother or baby is food-intolerant, extra care should be taken with the mother's diet—see treatment plan B or for more detail, earlier sections of this book.

4. PREVENTION OF DIARRHOEAL DISEASE

1. In pregnancy, eat a good balanced diet, avoiding your food allergens and avoiding 'binges' on any one food. Do not smoke; limit your alcohol intake; limit refined carbohydrates and avoid artificial sweeteners such as sorbitol, which can cause diarrhoea.

2. Breast-feed your baby exclusively from birth for the first 6 months. Practical advice about how to maximize your chances of succeeding at this is in Chapter 12.

3. Breast-feed your baby well into his second year or beyond. The immunological boost your milk supplies will help him resist bacterial and viral disease, and also help him cope with dietary and inhalant intolerances (if any). While breast-feeding, do not smoke or food binge.

4. From 6 months of age begin giving other good foods in very small quantities at first, and one at a time. Some babies may need other food earlier than 6 months; others thrive on breast milk alone for months yet. If the baby is healthy, happy, and gaining weight adequately, other food should be seen as unnecessary unless the mother needs to begin weaning.

5. Always observe basic rules of hygiene in cooking and caring for baby. Even where a safe water supply and plenty of fresh food is

available, children need to be taught to wash their hands before meals, after playing with animals, or after going to the toilet. And of course any food utensils must be kept clean. Obsessive expensive cleanliness elsewhere in the house, using lots of highly advertised germicides is largely a waste of time. No amount of chemical mix in his bath will prevent a baby from coming into contact with millions of bacteria and viruses—so keep a sense of perspective about hygiene. Safe food handling and storage is essential, though.

6. Avoid unnecessary medication; and where it is necessary, ask your doctor about the possible effects of the drug he has prescribed on the gut. If they prove to be severe, contact the doctor immediately to see if a change is possible. Beware of 'colic' medicines—one of their most active ingredients is alcohol. (If you want to give this to your baby, a few drops of brandy in warm water is probably less damaging than the highly coloured and flavoured kiddie recipes.) Some of these medicines have recently been withdrawn from sale because of possible problems (see p. 90).

Even if the technological know-how and the social organization is available, re-accelerating progress in child health depends upon the will to do so. In some nations, political will can be stimulated by national and international advocacy. Research and publicity, for example, can help to get across the message that simple diarrhoea is the major killer of children in most countries . . . and that a government committed to be greatest health of the greatest number at the lowest possible cost would certainly give more priority to oral rehydration salts than to heart-transplant technology.

UNICEF; *The state of the world's children*, p. 24. (1982).

17

Home testing for food intolerance

1. BEFORE YOU BEGIN

(a) Provocation testing and elimination diets all require considerable thought and organization. It is a family matter; it will only work with the full co-operation of everyone involved at home and away from home. Make sure that everyone understands every aspect of what to do and what not to do.

(b) Decide how you want to proceed—as quickly as possible, or as gently as possible. Pregnant and lactating women, and hypersensitive or very young children, should not be subject to extremes of dietary change or challenge. Adults who have had cardiac or respiratory symptoms need to take care too.

(c) Think about the option of a medically supervised fast or chemically defined diet[1] and testing in hospital, if you want answers in a hurry. It ought to be safer that way, although Rippere's experience was disturbing (see Bibliography). Of course it may be expensive if not on the NHS, and will not be a fun holiday. But for compulsive food addicts, behaviourally disturbed older children, and severely affected patients, it can be the best method. Adults with serious medical conditions such as diabetes, heart disease, and so on ought not to experiment with diet without medical supervision. In fact, I am assuming that you have recently had a medical check-up and the doctor has ruled out the possibility of other causes of your symptoms.

(d) Remember that you are individual. Look at any diet list and vary it according to your own knowledge. If you eat a great deal of any permitted food, or cannot do without one, suspect it as an allergen and omit it, or omit it if symptoms persist on the diet. Add in 'safe' fruits and vegetables that you have never eaten in excess.

(e) After four or five days elimination you often become hypersensitive to an allergen. Even small quantities at that time could cause a severe reaction. Make sure your children understand this, and avoid accidental or deliberate exposure.

(f) Many allergists suggest that you get a chemist to mix two parts of sodium bicarbonate with one part of potassium bicarbonate and keep this in the cupboard to help relieve symptoms. The dose for an adult is two teaspoons in a glass of water, followed by a second glass of water. (Ordinary sodium bicarbonate can also be used, but the above mixture is preferable.) This may be repeated in several hours if need be, but should not be used habitually or daily by adults, and not at all for infants or those whose doctors have advised against the use of a bicarbonate. (Ask if you are unsure.) Bicarbonate seems harmless enough, but it is not (see p. 137). And everyone is urging us to restrict our sodium intake. So if you use this remedy, do so with care.

The dose should be scaled down according to bodyweight for children: for example a 20 kg child should get one-third to one-quarter the adult dose. They say this works best at the first sign of trouble, rather than when symptoms are severe. A commercial alkali salts mixture is also available. In every case where you increase the body's mineral load, you *MUST* drink more water to keep your kidneys from being overloaded. This is essential if you have had any urinary or kidney problems (see Kilmartin).

2. WHAT FOODS DO YOU SUSPECT FIRST?

1. Foods that you actively dislike, and have 'because they are good for you'. Many women can't bear milk plain, but eat cheese instead, or cook with it, or have it in processed foods. Egg is another common suspect here.
2. Foods that you love, and eat lots of, or eat every day without fail. (More than 300–600 ml of milk for adults is excessive.)
3. Foods that you eat to 'pick you up', 'give you a lift'. Coffee, tea, cocoa, alcoholic beverages, other drugs and smokes, are the obvious suspects here—but any food that you eat regularly or 'don't feel right' without.
4. Foods that you know you were given as a very young baby—cows' milk, cereal, orange juices, but also fish (Hypol, cod liver oil).
5. Foods that grandma binged on while carrying *you*.

6. Foods that you remember making you sick as a child, or that you actively disliked but were made to eat.

7. Foods that your family is now eating which were not a part of your traditional racial diet. Migrants may have special problems in adapting to new foods as adults.

Is there anything left that is safe to eat??

Start with the most obvious suspects—remember that you may only have to eliminate a few major villains to be symptom-free.

For your baby,

1. all the above, plus
2. foods that you binged on in pregnancy and lactation.

3. DURING AN ELIMINATION PERIOD

(a) Don't be surprised if during the first 4–5 days you feel worse—tired, depressed, nervous, sleepless, confused with headaches or food cravings. Remember, the addict always has withdrawal symptoms; this possibility is acknowledged in the RCP/BNF Joint Report.[2] So hang on—it will pass and you will feel much better. If desperate, a tiny amount of an allergen may improve how you feel—but you must stay on the diet that much longer.

(b) Stay on the diet for at least two totally clear weeks—some would say up to a month, but for this you need to have your diet checked by a nutritionist, or be given professional advice about supplementation with minerals, trace elements, and vitamins.

4. REINTRODUCING FOODS

1. Never test a food unless you are feeling well. If you had a headache before the test and it gets worse after, you won't know the cause.

2. A good time to test is about 3 hours after breakfast. For school-children, afternoon tea time is probably the best: they are at home if immediate symptoms develop and delayed reaction will probably be evident before school the next day. However, if you can't

afford disturbed nights, keep the child home and test in the morning.

3. If you have no symptoms within 24 hours, add the test food back into your diet—that is don't eat it too often or too much.

4. Begin with the least suspect fruit and vegetables, leaving the most common allergens till later on. This means that you widen your diet as rapidly as possible, and so are less likely to develop new intolerances by eating too much of the same food.

5. Reintroduce one food at a time, at intervals of 5–6 days, to allow delayed reactions time to show up.

6. If you have a strong reaction to any food, wait for days if need be before introducing another.

7. Never test foods on yourself or an infant when you are isolated—without car, telephone, etc. Some reactions can be life-threatening without adrenaline and hospital care.

8. Keep full records of all testing and encourage the children to report infringements. (If you get cross about it, they probably won't!) These written records become invaluable when discussing the matter with your GP.

9. If you still feel unsure of procedure, read Rapp (*Allergies and Your Family*), pp. 144–156, or wait till you have found a helpful allergist. Make sure that your doctor has carefully read the material on diets in the RCP/BNF Report. Another book to recommend to him is that produced by the team at Addenbrooke's Hospital, Cambridge: *The allergy diet*, by Workman, Hunter, and Alun Jones.

5. WHAT TO DO?

(a) **The slow and gentle approach**

Simply keep a detailed diary of all that you eat and your state of health. For a child, record everything he eats, especially for the day of, *and the day before*, any symptoms. (Reactions may be immediate, or delayed—or both.) The RCP/BNP Joint Report stated that a diet diary should usually be kept over a period of 7 days but, if your life is not routine, you may need to keep a diet diary for a longer period.

Once you have built up a food diary, look at it for suspects. Then eliminate one or two of these at a time, and note changes (if any)

Food for thought

in well-being. This will be a slow and confusing business, because of the endless variations in your body's tolerance level *and* allergen load. However, over time some clarity will emerge. The diary must be complete—all food, drugs, and other possibly relevant information, such as emotional traumas, exposure to inhalants (for example changing the beds), visiting grandparents, change in exercise patterns, and so on.

(b) The single food test

Although a single food intolerance is probably rare, identifying and removing one major excitant may result in sufficient improvement for some people. The key to this is the hypersensitive period that developed at 4–5 days. What follows is one doctor's guide (his patients are adult of course).

Guide to challenging for food allergy at home

The principle of this test is to avoid the food in all its forms, and then try and provoke your symptoms by a good feed of the food in question. It is vital that the food should be totally avoided. Partial avoidance is not good enough, and if you make a mistake and have some of the forbidden food you must go back to the beginning again.

The food should be avoided in all its forms for 5 days, be it the food itself or when present in cooking or in any other form. In the case of milk this includes:

1. Milk from the bottle or carton
2. Powdered milk
3. Tinned milk
4. Derivatives of milk, e.g. yoghurt and cheese
5. Milk in cooking such as cakes and milk Vienna bread.

Once TOTAL abstinence from the food has been observed for 5 days, on the 6th day a large portion of the food is eaten *by itself* on an empty stomach, i.e. 3 hours after the previous meal. A good time is 11 a.m. after a light breakfast. If no symptoms are observed within the subsequent one hour, a further half portion is taken to act as a 'kicker dose'. Symptoms should be watched for and noted in the succeeding 24 hours.

If you feel you have a positive result to the challenge feed, you should always repeat the test.

Please notify this surgery of the results of all tests, either positive or negative.

146

Home testing for food intolerance

Should you get a marked reaction which distresses you, it can be relieved by drinking a glass of water containing two teaspoons of bicarbonate of soda, followed by two further glasses of plain water.

(For children this would have to be scaled down according to body weight.)

This procedure can be very dangerous, of course. Do not try it with a baby and note all previous cautions. It is best to have a well-informed friend in the house should you decide to try this.

Remember that 'a large portion' of the food means different things for different people. If your baby screams with colic when you have enough milk to whiten your coffee—though many intolerant mums can't take coffee either—it's not a good idea to drink half a litre to test. Use your common sense and knowledge of *your* degree of sensitivity.

Learn to recognize the early warning signs of a reaction. They are unique to you. One child of 6 notices that he 'feels funny' in the head and stomach initially—at which time his normal temperature (36.4°) has risen slightly (37.1°, or 'normal'). Often he has a slight sniff, or sneezes. In a short while his mouth is 'itchy'; temperature 37.6°. Within another half hour it will rise to 38° or more and he will have fleeting pains in odd places—unless given 250 mg paracetomol (plain tablet, no syrups) or some bicarbonate. Once you have established *personal* normal temperature and pulse rate (see Coca's book, listed in the Bibliography) these physiological markers can be very useful in confirming that an intolerant response is underway. This child also needs to go to the toilet within a couple of hours—stools are loosish and offensive. For a more detailed account, see Case History No. 1

(c) The elimination diet

Removing one food and substituting another may make no real difference to symptoms. (It commonly happens that milk is replaced by orange juice, and the person turns out in the end to be intolerant of both.) The principle of the elimination diet is to remove as many likely food excitants as possible, then to reintroduce them one at a time, noting changes that coincide.

Elimination diets vary enormously and are, as the RCP/BNF Joint Report puts it, 'necessarily arbitrary'.[3] Some allergists suggest the elimination of all but fruits, vegetables, and water, on the

Food for thought

grounds that the human body is best adapted to these over its evolutionary history. Most agree that common high-protein foods, refined carbohydrates, and chemically active foods like tea and coffee, should all go. Some urge the avoidance of 'natural' foods containing salicylates, and care with everything from aspirin to toothpaste. All would prefer the patient to have been tested for likely suspects first; all take it for granted that the patient will have stopped smoking and using other potent chemicals. Most books on allergies contain suggested elimination diets, so if this one seems to include all the foods you have binged on, find another. As we've said—there are no magically safe foods.

Elimination diets are not designed to be nutritionally adequate over a long period, so don't stay on one for too long. Most people will have begun to improve in the first two weeks, although the RCP/BNF Joint Report acknowledges that some people may take up to 3 weeks to show improvement.[4] This is the commonest criticism of the book, that no matter how many times you are told not to stay on unbalanced diets, you the reader are silly enough to do just that. I hope my belief in your common sense is justified. This is particularly important for children, whose growth must be constantly monitored. One study showed that 15 of 108 children on elimination diets prior to referral to one specialist, showed frank failure to thrive.[5] (Mind you, they may already have been malnourished before being placed on the diet—presumably this was not just done capriciously but in an attempt to resolve long-standing problems. Such a possibility is not raised by those who criticize elimination diets.)

If your symptoms are relieved during the period of the diet, try to have the identity of the allergens confirmed by controlled challenges under medical supervision. This is a risky business, and you do need some further reassurance that the tedium of dietary change is really justified, or your compliance with your diet will fall away after the initial enthusiasm. But, if being tested by a doctor, make sure he is aware of all that the RCP/BNF Joint Report says about challenge testing. Not many doctors recognize that, 'for those whose symptoms are slow to develop, a disguised purée preparation may have to be given over a period of 2 weeks',[6] that measuring sub-clinical changes may be necessary; that withdrawal symptoms may occur; and so on. Many doctors still give standardized doses of common allergens in ways which do not

148

Home testing for food intolerance

replicate the patient's normal exposure to the foods, then write-off the patient as suffering from psychosomatic symptoms when he (or even more commonly, she) fails to respond. This is rightly criticized by Dr Morrow Brown in an excellent chapter of Freed's book, *Health hazards of milk.*

Elimination diet (sample supplied by a GP)

You may have:

Lamb, rice, tapioca, spinach, celery, sweet potato, lettuce, beetroot, artichoke, carrot, pears, cherries, pineapple, salt, pepper, parsley, olive oil, sunflower oil, kosher or vitaquel margarine, malt vinegar, water, percolated coffee (weak, and only if you're not a coffee addict, or breast-feeding, or pregnant).

NAME ....

FOOD	DAY Date	SYMPTOMS (0 to 3)						
Lamb								
Rice								
Lettuce								
Carrot								

MEDICATIONS
tabs per (   ) day

(symptoms: 0—nil, 1—mild, 2—moderate, 3—severe)

Note
1. Fruit should be fresh. Preserved may be used provided the container carries a notice definitely excluding preservatives and colouring matter. Avoid too much food stored in plastic or metal.
2. Try some of the attached recipes.
3. You may *not* have:
★ any foods or drinks not listed above
★ milk, tea, soft drinks including colas, alcoholic drinks
★ sweets, lollies, chewing gum
★ any medications or tablets not prescribed by your doctor

Oils and margarines may contain anti-oxidants, which may not be tolerated by the chemical-sensitive.

(d) After identifying allergens

1. Decide whether total avoidance is practical and worthwhile, that is whether the difficulties of eliminating the food are outweighed by difficulties the food causes you. For children, total avoidance (at least for a year or more) is probably advisable, but for adults this should be a personal decision.

2. If avoidance involves major dietary changes, work out substitutes for foods omitted, then get your diet checked out by a nutritionist. Invest in some allergy cookbooks.

3. Periodically review the family diet every few months. If calcium or other vitamin or mineral supplements are prescribed by a nutritionist or doctor, ask for hypoallergenic ones—like most medications, supplements are full of potent chemical excitants. Remember this when any drug is prescribed. If patients ask for hypoallergenic drugs the companies will provide them, eventually. Note any adverse reactions and ask your chemist to send a report to the authorities responsible for monitoring drug reactions.

4. As soon as problem foods are identified, let your children's teachers and other children's parents know. Explain the basic problem thoroughly; perhaps lend them this book. To have to refuse 'normal' foods and perhaps also opt out of some school activities can be an enormous strain for a child—he needs support. The very allergic child should not be given dusty or smelly jobs to do, and all food provided at school must be scrutinized. (Don't forget the kindergarten glass of milk!) Teachers should know what symptoms spell trouble, or at least, be prepared to believe the child, who is almost always right about his problems, once he has been educated.

Brace yourself for some hard times though. Until other children's problems are recognized for what they are, you will amost certainly be seen as neurotic by at least some teachers. Your child's headaches or nosebleeds will be thought to be attention-seeking behaviour, especially if they become frequent. He or she may be deeply hurt or angered by the teacher's lack of comprehension. In fact it may be the schoolroom itself which is causing the child's problems—foods are easily controlled, but many schools expose children to a wide variety of inhalant excitants, chiefly chemicals. Look into that if the child complains of aches and pains at school. In my son's case it turned out to be the paper, treated by a spirit duplicator, which gave him headaches, though I suspect that his teacher still believes that he 'just isn't used to loud noise'. She had never heard me yelling at the kids, of course, and, being unmarried, had a slightly unreal view of the noise levels of a household of five. Some children have problems with teachers who smoke or use fly spray in the room too. And natural gas heating causes many headaches and wheezes.

5. Remember that the first months of adjusting to a new diet, new shopping, and cooking habits, and so on are very demanding—but that once you get used to the new framework of your life it will become second nature. Change *is* hard—it is stressful for everyone—so try to work as a family in all of this. If you can interest some friends, so much the better; you need support. Joining, or starting, an allergy self-help group is an excellent idea. By pooling funds you can acquire a much wider range of useful literature, and there is no substitute for other people's ideas and interest.

In fact, so important is it that you do not act alone, but get in touch with other parents, that I am very tempted to omit the sample elimination diet and recipes in future editions. As it is, they are barely adequate, and groups like AAA have much better selections. So once again, do join, and ask for their recipes—but remember that such groups do not run on air, and at least cover costs, if you can. Other books, with better elimination diets, are listed in the Bibliography section; I particularly like Workman *et al*.

DIET RECIPES

Lamb stock
Lamb bones with some meat
6 cups water
2 sticks celery, sliced
2 sweet potatoes, sliced
salt, pepper

Place all ingredients into a saucepan and bring to boil. Simmer 1 hour. Cool and skim of fat.

Food for thought

Beetroot soup
1 quantity lamb stock
4 beetroot—sliced or cubed

Simmer beetroot in stock for
$\frac{3}{4}$–1 hour, add salt and pepper
to taste. Sprinkle with chopped
parsley and serve.

Vegetable soup
1 quantity lamb stock
$\frac{1}{2}$ small bunch spinach, shredded
2 sweet potatoes, cubed
2 sticks celery, sliced
salt, pepper

Add vegetables and seasoning
to stock and cook gently until
vegetables are soft.

Main courses

Risotto—4 portions
4 oz rice (patna)
1 oz oil
salt
1 pint of water
2 cups chopped cooked lamb
pineapple pieces

Wash rice; heat oil. Stir in rice.
Add stock and seasoning. Put
on lid and cook gently until
soft. Add chopped meat and
pineapple pieces and cook
further 5–10 minutes.

Sweet and sour lamb—2
  portions
$\frac{1}{2}$ lb lamp chops
oil to fry lamb
1 teacup water
pineapple pieces
2 dessertsp. vinegar
$\frac{1}{2}$ teaspoon salt

Fry lamb in hot oil; brown
quickly. Drain off excess oil.
Add all ingredients and bring to
boil. Simmer until meat and
vegetables are tender—approx.
$1\frac{1}{4}$ hrs

Meat sauce
$1\frac{1}{2}$ lb minced lamb
1 cup chopped celery
Fry meat; brown well. Add
celery.

Add water and simmer till
cooked.
Thicken with rice flour. Serve
over rice.

Rice salad
3 cups cooked rice
1 cup cooked lamb pieces (left
over from roast)
1 cup chopped celery
French dressing

Mix all ingredients, chill well
and serve.

Home testing for food intolerance

Fried rice
1 lb rice, 3 cups cold water, salt

Wash rice and drain off water. Cover with 3 cups of cold water. Add salt, cover with lid. Bring to boil on medium heat and cook 20 mins.

2 cups chopped celery
½ cup shredded spinach (cooked)
1 lb diced cooked lamb
chopped parsley

Gently fry celery; add meat and spinach. Add rice and fry gently. Mix well. Serve hot.

Lamb stew with rice
1½ lb lamb
rice flour
salt, pepper
1 tablespoon oil
2 sticks celery
1 tablespoon parsley
2 tablespoons uncooked rice
1 pint water
2 sweet potatoes, cubed

Cut meat into cubes, coat with flour, salt and pepper. Brown in hot oil and place into casserole; add water to pan then add celery and potatoes. Stir until boiling then pour over meat in casserole and cover tightly and cook slowly in a moderate oven for approx. 2 hours.

Cream of celery soup
1 oz oil
1 pint lamb stock
2 tablespoons rice flour
salt and pepper
2 cups cooked celery

Warm oil, add flour and seasoning. Stir till smooth. Add ½ pint lamb stock and stir till smooth. Add remaining stock. Stir in celery (sliced) and ½ sweet potato and some fresh celery.

Rice pancakes
1 cup cooked rice
1 cup rice flour
½ cup water
diced pears or apricots or cherries
pinch salt

Mix flour, water and salt. Add rice and fry in hot oil, top with fruit.

Fruit rice pudding
1 cup stewed pineapple, (tinned is all right), apricot or pears (or a mixture)

1 cup cooked rice
¾ cup water

Place drained fruit in oiled dish. Cover with drained rice, pour water over rice. Bake in a moderate oven (400 °F) for 45 mins.

Food for thought

Rice bread

8 oz (250g) rice flour
½ teaspoon sodium bicarb.
1 teaspoon cream of tartar
2 tablespoons oil
½ teaspoon salt
6 oz (180 ml) water

Sift dry ingredients. Add water and oil, beating with fork. Put into oiled 1lb loaf tin. Bake in top of oven at 375 °F for approx. 30 mins. Loaf should rebounce to touch.

Many more recipes will be found in Rapp, Conrad, etc. Write to AAA (p. 193) or to Wholefood, (p. 197) for a price list.

18

About 'allergy' for people aged 7–17

By now you know that there are things that you eat, breathe, or touch which cause changes in the way your body behaves. This is a real nuisance, and you may feel annoyed that this had to happen to you, because it makes you different from other kids—who probably tease you about it sometimes. It doesn't seem fair. There are a few things you should know.

1. First of all, this problem is very common. Probably some of your schoolfriends suffer from it too, but their parents have not found out why they get ill, or are slow to learn, or behave badly.

2. It is not as bad a problem as other sorts of handicap—because it is one that *you* can manage yourself most of the time. If you're sensible, you won't have to spend a lot of time feeling rotten, and can live a normal life.

3. It is an awful problem for your parents, who probably spent much time and energy finding out what was wrong with you (and them, sometimes). Other people still make them feel bad about it because those other people don't know enough. Your parents need your help.

4. If you were a rotten kid for years before your parents found out why, that will have made a difference to how you and they get on. In the same way, if your parents were badly affected for years, they may have found it hard to be as loving to you as they probably wanted to be. How you get on now is your responsibility as well as theirs. If you have any grudges about how they treated you, talk about it and try to listen to their side. Ask them to tell you what they had to go through.

5. It is your body, no-one else's. Your parents should give you whatever information you need to avoid problems. But it is not their job to see that you *do* avoid them. If you want these things despite the consequences, it's your body that suffers. When you're young you don't think about what the consequences will be next

week, much less in a few years. But you do need to. Play around with these problems and you could kill yourself. More and more young adults are dying of asthma these days. No-one can predict which time a major mistake could prove to be just too much for your body to cope with. So if you do want to break the rules and have a binge, or ignore your medication, don't do it unless there's someone around who knows what to do if you're badly affected.

6. Get used to the idea that cigarettes and grog are just not things you will be able to handle and stay healthy. Try to avoid being sucked in by those who are too ignorant or stupid to realize what harm they are doing their bodies. Learn to see advertising as a cynical attempt to rip you off.

7. Your parents can look after what happens at home, but they can't control what happens at school, at other people's places, and all the other places you will be. If you feel bad at, or after being at, any other place you will have to do your own detective work. Learn to notice all the tiny indications your body makes—that slight sniffle, or itch, or headache (though these are often delayed reactions too). It is *your* body—no-one else knows what it feels like to live in it, so no-one else can know what's normal for you.

8. Don't be surprised or upset if teachers, or other parents, or anyone lets you know that they think this is simply hypochondria (which means you think you are ill when you are not). They are just ignorant—they can't help that. Give them something to read about all this. If they are still not convinced, don't waste time arguing. If they should try to make you do something that you know will make you ill—like dusty work, or work with chemicals (glues, duplicators, etc.) refuse politely—ask to speak to the head teacher if need be. But most adults will be quite understanding once it has all been explained to them.

9. Try not to let other kids know that teasing upsets you. It will probably make them worse.

10. Even when you've been really well for long periods of time, you can't afford to completely forget your earlier problems. It pays to be careful with your diet when you know you are going to be under any stress or in times of altered hormone functioning—for example, before exams, when due to play energetic sport, before

and during menstruation or in puberty, in times of family crisis, and so on.

11. Remember that foods can be just as addictive as drugs, and the habit just as hard to break. Don't feel bad about yourself if you find that you keep failing. Adults find it hard to quit smoking, after all.

12. If there are things you can do to help yourself—like taking medication or vitamins—then do it. Don't cause extra family problems by having to be nagged about everything. *Taking responsibility for your own body and your own behaviour is what growing up is all about.*

This all sounds like a sermon. It is not meant to be. I am writing this because I have dealt with a lot of families and know that what is a simple dietary problem can lead to all kinds of unhappiness where kids and parents can't work together. For your own sake, and your family's, do your best.

19

About allergy for grandparents and other assorted child-care-givers

This too is your problem and your responsibility. Even if it may sometimes seem to contradict some of your cherished beliefs, you must take seriously what the parents of a child tell you about his sensitivities to foods or chemicals. When you do not, you create enormous and very basic problems for that family unit. Tensions between parents—'no, we won't go to your parents because they disregard my requests not to give sweets and *you* won't be around tomorrow to cope with the consequences?' Tensions between parents and child—'but grandma lets me have milk and she says it's good for me.' Tensions between you and parents—'but if I can't trust him not to sneak treats to the kids, or even to tell me when he has, how can we leave the kids there?'

If you care for the child or its parents, you will readily see that such tensions are damaging to everyone. Your role as a care-giver is to help that family unit cope with the myriad stresses of modern life—not to add to them. You should be supporting the parents in their most basic role, enabling them to feel more competent and confident—not undermining their confidence.

That does not mean there can be no disagreement or debate. But the ground rules for that must be:

(a) everything is out in the open, not muttered to sympathetic ears elsewhere.

(b) the parents' expressed will must prevail (within the bounds of reason!) They must be able to trust you to do as they ask or to tell them of any infringements.

If that seems impossible, it is probably better to decline to care for that particular child.

Grandparents especially are enormously important. 'One of the most cheering aspects of handling distribution of the books is to realize just how many caring, open-minded, intelligent older people have seen the relevance of this work to their children and grandchildren (or other family and friends). Many write ruefully of the realization that grandson's colic may have had more to do with their failed breast-feeding than with their daughter's parenting skills—for their daughter, reared on cows'/goats'/other milks, has

158

'Allergy' for grandparents and assorted child-care-givers

had food problems all her life. Many are already aware of the impact of foods upon themselves, and rejoice to find a book which 'makes my observations respectable', as one said.

As grandparents, you have seen fashions in infant rearing come and go. These new ideas may seem to be just another fad. The difference is that for the first time in history, researchers are looking scientifically at both the short- and long-term consequences of what we do to babies, for the first time we have the capacity to *begin* to analyse human milk and find out what ought to be in formulae. (Finding out how to put it there is another problem.) So if it seems like another fad when your daughter not only wants to breast-feed, but does so beyond whatever arbitrary age babies are 'supposed' to be breast-fed for, or does so in public—support her, whether you breast-or bottle-fed her. (If you did bottle-feed, realize that breast-fed babies are different—perhaps buy a book like *Breast is best*, as you're never too old to learn.) There is no need to feel guilty, even if it now seems that some things could have been done better—you did your best at the time. What you now have to do is help this new mother do *her* best, in the light of new information. Don't offer to take the baby for a weekend—but do encourage her to express enough milk and leave baby and her milk with you for an evening. Don't bribe toddler with forbidden foods—you'll find there are plenty of effective and permitted bribes—or rewards to reinforce positive behaviour, as they now say. If you think her ideas crazy, tell her so, but also assure her that because you care for her she can rely on you to do whatever is agreed. If, as you get older, it seems too difficult to organize alternative foods, etc. ask the parents to bring all the necessities with them. (Most usually do.)

In short, because the problem of food intolerance does create practical difficulties for families, they need your support and love more than ever. Don't let things get to this stage . . .

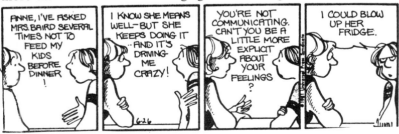

For Better, for Worse—Lynn Johnston.   © Alan Foley Pty. Ltd.

20

Some changes to work for

Parents who feel sufficiently strongly about these matters could do a great deal to bring about change. My December 1981 submission to the National Health and Medical Research Council spelt out some of the concerns parents raised. This was published in full in earlier editions, and copies are still available from me if people are interested. Most of those concerns have been incorporated in the text of this edition, and the submission has been deleted to make room for additional material.

It was included initially to make the point that the key to real improvement is always 'political' influence. Not in any narrow sense of party politics, which parent groups do well to keep clear of—their causes are beyond politics in that sense. But decisions about how a society's resources are to be allocated, what money is to be spent on what research, or education, or advertising programmes—these are all political decisions. An organization's decision to act as a consumer lobby is a political decision—and so too is an organization's decision NOT to act as a consumer lobby. It is impossible to be apolitical when seeking change. A decision to never ruffle the medical profession's feather for instance, is as much political as the decision to speak openly and honestly, even if that may entail the odd controversy. Those who deliberately choose the former must accept some responsibility for the unchanged status quo, just as those who choose the latter must run the risk of hardening intransigent attitudes. There is obviously room for both approaches in society, and organizations can adopt different attitudes as their power base and their leadership changes. It would be silly, for example, for a group of half a dozen undereducated people to challenge the status quo without any real backing from medical authorities. On the other hand, if that group represented thousands, had a proven success rate, and a mountain of research data and clinical experience validating its position, it would be in a totally altered position, and new strategies would be possible. Of course they will continue the primary task of putting plasters on problems created by the status quo, but such a body

Some changes to work for

could also be exploring ways of altering the status quo, by working co-operatively with those who have power to change it—even by calmly and publicly exposing the damaging realities which make band aids necessary.

So people who want change need to organize. Parents need to get together, form their local self-help groups, then make common cause with all the other self help groups affected directly and indirectly by these matters. We are not talking about acts of God or natural disasters, but about man-made illness which is very largely preventable and manageable, and which affects almost everyone in this society. Let's get it fixed! Some places to begin:

1. Attention to allergic history in pregnancy

(a) Clear and specific dietary guidelines for mothers-to-be, with simple explanation of the importance of compliance for her baby—to avoid *in utero* sensitization.[1]

(b) Clear explanation of the unique importance of breast-feeding, particularly for the baby of an allergic family, and the need to avoid any complementary feeding in the first weeks and months. The mother should be put in touch with local support groups such as the National Childbirth Trust, the Association of Breastfeeding Mothers, etc. (see pp. 198–9).

(c) Definite follow-up to the hospital when mother books in, noting her allergic history and need for care with baby.

2. Abolition of the 'comp' bottle in maternity hospitals

The comp bottle should be replaced by human milk complements (given by dropper) in the few cases where this is really necessary. This will entail a complete change from 'schedule' to *ad libitum* feeding, which is possible only when baby 'rooms in' during the day at least. Night feeding should become the rule for mothers, although nurses can make that only a minor interruption by bringing the child to the mother when it first wakes. As in Finland, the major factor needed for successful breast-feeding is probably the better education of mid-wives—both in the art of managing lactation and the importance of breast-feeding. Some nurses are even unaware that 'formulae' are cows' milk-based, so successfully have the companies promoted their 'humanized' products. As in Sweden, all human babies should receive only human milk in hospital. Can you imagine a prize foal being fed cows' milk in its first days of life?

Food for thought

3. *Better nutritional advice and follow-up in the post-partum period*

Specific guidelines about introducing other foods—long before the mother actually begins to. (Many current recommendations cannot be justified by research findings.) Nutrition education should begin in the primary schools, and the promotion of breast-feeding should be an integral part of it. A better deal for working mothers—longer maternity leave, provision for nursing breaks, facilities at work for very young babies.

4. *A national campaign*

To educate everyone from tinies to grandparents about the advantages of breast-feeding, and the need to delay introduction of other foods. The establishment of milk banks (or a human milk industry?) to supply milk for babies whose mothers cannot produce enough ... Even, as in New York and Sweden, legislation to guarantee the availability of human milk. Governments must accept a real share of the responsibility for such a campaign. It's not good enough to leave it to enthusiastic amateurs. Such a campaign must not simply promote the idea that breast is best—most women already accept this and attempt to breast-feed. The campaign needs to include better education of professionals, new research into the problems of breast-feeding management, changes in hospital policies, changes in socioeconomic and cultural practices and attitudes which make continued breast-feeding difficult. To push breast-feeding without this concerted strategy is to invite failure—and to make mothers feel even more guilty, more of a failure, than if they believed formula to be the same as breast milk. The Canadian and Brazilian campaigns have much to say to the rest of the world.

5. *More, rather than less, recognition of the increasing role of allergy in the nation's health costs*

This should be accompanied by more support for parents who by dietary manipulation are preventing costly illness. Diagnostic and preventive medicine of this kind is far cheaper than hospitalization, intensive therapy, and drugs. Goats' and soy milks and any other dietary aids should be more readily available. Allergy clinics should exist in all major centres. All of these things are the subject of cutbacks at the moment. However, it has recently become poss-

Some changes to work for

ible within Australia to claim some of your expenses as a tax deducation. This would be worth testing in the UK.

6. Better food labelling and better food

Like Australia, the UK has regulations requiring labelling of additives. However, to decipher a list of ingredients is not always easy. A booklet translating the serial numbers, and explaining the new labelling regulations is available from, MAFF, Publications Unit, Lion House, Willowburn Trading Estate, Alnwick, Northumberland NE66 2PF. But manufacturers need to know the extent of the problems they are inadvertently and sometimes unnecessarily causing. Who really wants bright yellow margarine once he knows that the colour is just there for asethetic reasons? Why put preservatives into pasteurized fruit juices? Write and tell the manufacturer why you cannot buy his food. Commercial interests respond very rapidly to financial incentives.

7. Stringent control of advertising

This should be especially for infant foods, drugs, and drinks. Despite the rhetoric of corporate responsibility, it has been concerted international action by consumers and professionals which has brought about the WHO Code of Marketing of Breastmilk Substitutes. But I would like to urge you to see that the Code is more than a piece of paper by reporting violations of it (here and overseas) to the groups which are monitoring the situation around the world. See p. 166. As a recent visitor to many UK hospitals, I was shocked by the constant presence of Cow & Gate, and other formula manufacturers' goods in maternity wards.

Changes in these and other areas will come about only if each of us exerts what little power we possess as citizens, as taxpayers, as patients, as parents, and as consumers. Do not suffer in silence—put pen to paper.

To change behaviour is always difficult, but trends in infant feeding over the last two years show that it can be done, and in a relatively short time too. A national campaign in which the media play a big part and in which a less desirable commodity is made difficult to obtain is likely to produce results.

F. Brindlecombe, *Public Health* **91** 117, (1977).

21

International change: and appeal and a programme from UNICEF

As part of the world community, Britain is called upon to implement UNICEF's 'child revolution'. While the results may be more dramatic in countries without clear water supplies, the UNICEF measures are very relevant to every family particularly the growing numbers of 'socially disadvantaged'. And those of us with greater resources have a moral obligation to do what we can to help, nationally and internationally, in this basic health programme. Hence I am here reprinting in full an article from *The Lancet* (1983, *i*, 55) which summarizes the UNICEF appeal.[1]

The obviously starving child is the extreme tip of the mountain of malnutrition. Most of the 40 000 children who die daily throughout the world succumb to infections superimposed on the seldom visible undernourishment caused by repeated bouts of diarrhoea. The 1982–83 report[1] by UNICEF's executive director, James P. Grant, proffers four strategies by which to break the cycle of malnutrition and disease. In his estimate, the lives of 20 000 children a day could be saved by these relatively inexpensive measures.

Oral rehydration therapy (ORT) permits the mother to make up her own oral rehydration solution (one teaspoonful of salt to eight teaspoonfuls of sugar per litre of boiled, cooled water) or to buy cheap packets of ready-made salts and administer the mixture in her own home to the child dehydrated by diarrhoea. The discovery that adding glucose to a salt solution increased the body's rate of absorption of fluid by 2500 per cent has meant that dehydrated children seldom have to be treated intravenously by trained personnel—if such facilities even exist. In Narangwal, India, the death-rate among young children has been halved by community workers using oral rehydration salts and penicillin. Grant writes: 'The need for ORT is clear, the technology is known, the means of dissemination are available. The receptiveness of parents has been demonstrated. The cost is small. And only an inexcusable lack of national and international will can now prevent the bringing of its benefits to the vast majority of children in need.

The development of more stable and effective vaccines and the reduction in their cost has made the second plan of *mass initial and booster immunization* feasible. Measles, diphtheria, tetanus, whooping-cough, poliomyelitis, and tuberculosis account for about a third of all child

164

deaths. The malnourished child is susceptible to disease and disease pro-
vokes malnutrition.

The third proposal is the promotion of *breast-feeding*. UNICEF sponsored a 4-year study of over 10 000 newborn infants in a hospital in the
Philippines. After 2 years, its director of paediatrics declared: 'I closed the
door of the nursery to the milk companies. We stopped giving our babies
the standard dose of infant formula. Down came the colourful posters and
calendars. In their place, we hung the 'baby-killer' posters which show an
emaciated baby inside a dirty feeding bottle. Everything that was condu-
cive to bottle-feeding was removed not only from the nurseries but from
everywhere else in the hospital. I myself rejected samples and donations
from the milk companies'. Over the next 2 years, the incidence of infection, diarrhoea, and death among the newborns fell. In Papua New
Guinea, where legislation which accords with the subsequent World
Health Organisation code of marketing for breast-milk substitutes, was
passed in 1977, the percentage of bottle-fed infants fell from 35 per cent
to 12 per cent and serious undernourishment was reduced from 11 per
cent to 4 per cent.

The final weapon in the fight against malnutrition is the mass distribution of simple carboard *weight charts*. Mothers are taught to enter the
monthly weight of her child and compare it to an expected rise in weight
so that any failure to gain is clearly visible, and corrected, where possible,
by extra food. A depressing example of an actual child's development in
Central America is included in the report. The graph shows the continual
interruptions in weight gain by diseases after the cessation of breast-
feeding. At 18 months, the child weighed the same as he had done at 6
months.

As Grant emphasizes, a substantial drop in the perinatal and child
mortality rate does not produce a population boom: 'It is a conflict which
is dissolved by time. For when people become more confident that their
existing children will survive, they tend to have fewer births. That is the
principal reason why no nation has ever seen a significant and sustained
fall in its birth rate without first seeing a fall in its child death rate'. In
addition, the report suggests effectively targeted food subsidies (to the
malnourished children indicated by growth charts, for example), and the
fundamental services of clean water, sanitation, and basic literacy.

The business of improving the chances of vulnerable children has endless ramifications. UNICEF has concerned itself with just four simple
processes which depend for their efficacy on a network of education to
extend into the remotest areas of the world. The enthusiasm and hard
work of innumerable health and community workers is required to instil
knowledge of the simple remedies that can save children's lives.

The *Lancet's* account of the 1982–3 Grant report is a good summary, but lacks the impact of the Report itself. The 1982–3 report
ended by saying 'If the target (of halving the infant and child death
rate in the year 2000) is indeed laid by, then it means that the

number of children who die unnecessarily each year from now on will be the equivalent of the entire under-five population of the USA or the combined child populations of the UK France, West Germany, Italy, and Spain . . .

In a world distracted by so many deceptive and dangerous kinds of progress, we refuse to accept that such truly human and truly civilised progress as saving the lives and improving the health of the world's children should be abandoned at the first sign of difficulty. And we believe that if the political will can be found to seize the opportunities offered by recent social and scientific progress, then the goal of adequate food and health for the vast majority of the world's children need not be a dream deferred.'

How much will you be giving this year to overseas aid projects, or researchers working in these areas? And what will you do to tell others of UNICEF's goals? Or to put them into practice in Britain? The 1984 UNICEF Report also written by Grant, is even more direct in its demands:

The challenge of the children's revolution is . . . a challenge for both governments and people. And for those who might doubt what ordinary people can achieve in the service of such a cause, it is worth recollecting that it is movements which have enlisted the commitment and caught the imagination of people which have brought about some of the greatest political and social changes of our times—The movement for political independence in the Third World . . . for civil rights in the USA for the ending of unjust wars; for the protection of the environment, and for the rights of women.

If you read nothing else, write to UNICEF for a copy of the 1986 Report on the *State of the World's Children.*

THE WHO CODE OF MARKETING OF BREASTMILK SUBSTITUTES

One practical thing you can do is to monitor the observance of the WHO code of Marketing of Breastmilk Substitutes, wherever you are living. Before going any further, it may be as well to fill in some background to the controversy you have probably been aware of, surrounding International Baby Foods Action Network (IBFAN) and the Code.

International change

IBFAN was formed after the 1979 Geneva WHO/UNICEF joint meeting on infant and young child feeding. It is an umbrella group of consumer, religious, and international aid agencies such as Oxfam, the International Union of Consumer Organizations, the Interfaith Centre for Corporate Responsibility. Its international monitoring of violations of 'voluntary' industry restraints helped to bring about the WHO code. That Code is only a beginning—it represents a compromise between what aid agencies and other professionals wanted and what industry would accept. Violations continue and some industry instructions to employees have been stringently criticized as breaking the Code in spirit if not in strict legal terms. The Code is to be continually monitored and reassessed every two years.

Like Australia, neither Britain nor the USA has yet acted to adopt the WHO code in full. Countries with established infant formula industries usually agreed with the code 'in principle', but were reluctant or unable to put it into practice. The concerted lobbying of manufacturers persuaded the US Government to vote against the code—the only country to do so. In Britain the Food Manufacturers' Federation (FMF) produced their own version, a voluntary code which in many significant respects was weaker than the WHO code. The Government agreed to this, without adequate consultation of either medical or lay experts. The National Childbirth Trust has protested strongly, saying that the FMF code should be seen only as a beginning, and objecting to many of its provisions. Consumer groups in both countries refuse to accept less than the WHO code, and continue to press their governments to provide the minimum protection of the WHO code itself.

Governments in 'developed' countries commonly argue that the WHO code is not needed to protect their children; that sanitation and education standards are such that the problems common in poor countries are insignificant in developed ones. This really is nonsense. Every country has disadvantaged minorities. The current recession has led to enormous problems for such groups—and who can afford the expensive 'humanized' formulae when jobless? (One recent documentary on Australian television stated that in depressed areas US infant mortality rates were as high as in Third World countries.) In the USA, a remarkable document has been prepared by a national coalition of concerned groups. Entitled 'A petition to alleviate domestic infant formula

167

misuse and provide informed infant feeding choice' (cf. p. 229); it quite clearly shows the harm being done to children in the world's wealthiest nation. (In Australia we are working on a similar document.) If the economic outlook remains bleak, how many other families will have to find cheap or inadequate infant foods? As Dr Sai, chairman of the October 1979 WHO/UNICEF meeting, said, 'The talking has gone on long enough. It is time for action, based on that sense of moral outrage (*Lancet* (1980) **ii**, 258).

If you want parent groups of which you are a member to do more about this issue, write and tell them so.

WHAT YOU CAN DO? BE A CODEWATCHER

Read what follows and notify IBFAN of any violations. (Photocopy the following pages or write a letter— it doesn't matter.)

Have you noticed artificial baby milk, bottles, or teats advertised in magazines, newpapers, radio, TV, posters, etc?

Please tick: **Yes** ☐ **No** ☐ If yes, please describe the advertisement
● Brand name
● Month and year of advert
● Type of advertisement (TV? poster?)
● Location (which city? clinic? magazine?)
● Description of advertisement (written content, pictures)
● Any pictures of babies: use of words like 'humanized'?
Have you noticed any promotion of baby-milk direct to the public via special displays, price reductions, discount premiums, gifts, offers of free samples if you write?

Free gifts

Have you noticed baby booklets, brochures, bottle, clothing, posters, calendars, weighcards, wrist-bands or baby shows sponsored by baby-milk companies?

Please tick: **Yes** ☐ **No** ☐ If yes, please give details.
● Company name
● Type of gift (bottle? booklet?)
● Month and year of gift
● Where given (name of clinic, etc)

International change

● Description of gift/event* (given to whom? quantities? contents?)

Company agents

Do you know of employees of baby-milk companies that visit local hospitals, clinics, stores, health ministries?

Please tick: **Yes** □ **No** □ If yes, please give details.
● Which companies?
● Where do their agents visit?
● Number of visits per month
● Most recent date of visit
● Do doctors/nurses request such visits?
● Do the company agents talk with mothers?
● Do they have written permission from doctors to talk to mothers?

Samples

Do you know whether free samples of artificial baby-milk are donated to hospitals and clinics by companies?

Please tick: **Yes** □ **No** □ If yes, please detail recent donations.
● Which brand?
● How many samples per month?
● Do health staff give samples to mothers?
● Do health staff give samples to mothers?
● How much does each mother receive?
● What percentage of mothers receive free samples?
● Name and brief address of clinic/hospital
● Do hospital and manufacturer 'take steps to ensure that supplies [of donated formula] can be continued as long as the infants concerned need them'?

Influencing health personnel

A. *Do baby-milk companies give health workers written material?*

Please tick: **Yes** □ **No** □ If yes, please give details.
● Which company?
● Does the written mention superiority of breast-feeding?

Food for thought

- Mention hazards of bottle-feeding?
- Imply bottle-feeding is nearly equal to breast-feeding?

B. *Do you know of companies that give health workers free samples for their own babies?*

Please tick: **Yes** □ **No** □ If yes, please give details
- Which company?
- Month and year donated.
- Given to whom?
- Description of gift

C. *Do you know of baby-milk companies that give health workers personal gifts?*

Please tick: **Yes** □ **No** □ If yes, please give details
- Which company?
- Month and year donated
- Given to whom?
- Description of gift

D. *Do you know of baby-milk companies that provide money for research, travel, conferences, dinners medical equipment?*

Please tick: **Yes** □ **No** □ If yes, please give details
- Which company?
- Month and year donated
- Given to whom?
- Description of donation

Information and education

- What evidence have you seen that local and national governments have accepted their 'responsibility to ensure that *consistent* and *objective* information is provided on infant and young child feeding for use by families and those involved in the field of infant and young child nutrition'?
- Do *all* informational materials, 'whether written, audio, or visual, dealing with the feeding of infants . . . include clear information on the following points: (a) the benefits and superiority of breast-feeding; (b) maternal nutrition, and the preparation

170

for and maintenance of breast-feeding; (c) the negative effect on breast-feeding of introducing partial bottle-feeding; (d) the difficulty of reversing the decision not to breast-feed . . .'

● Do all such materials, where it is necessary to, include information about the proper use of infant formula, also 'the social and financial implications of its use; the health hazards of inappropriate foods or feeding methods; and, in particular, the health hazards of unnecessary or improper use of infant formula and other breast-milk substitutes'? Do such materials 'not use any pictures or text which may idealize the use of breast-milk substitutes'?

Optional

Your name _____

Organization _____

Address _____

_____

_____

Date _____

May your name be cited as a source of information?
Please tick: Yes ☐ No ☐
  * If possible, please send the original material, or a copy or a photo of it. International Baby Food Action will reimburse you for mailing costs of the example, if you request this.

Send your report to: Baby Milk Action Coalition, c/o Patti Rundall, 34 Blinco Grove, Cambridge, UK or War on Want, 467 Caledonian Road, London N7 9BE, and a copy to the National Childbirth Trust. For an excellent account of the history and content of the WHO code and the whole controversy, I cannot recommend too highly a La Leche League International tape, Who Supports the WHO Code? by K. Cravero. (Available from LLLI or Duplicord, 3S123 Route (59), Box 242, Warrenville, Illinois 60555, USA.)

PART 3

Miscellaneous

22

Case histories

I decided against incorporating these case histories (and hundreds of others) into the text because many professionals find anecdotes irritating. They are included not as proof, but by way of illustration. I therefore chose the most normal cases, rather than the most extreme, and limited the choice to families with whom I have had prolonged contact. However, I could not resist including the last letter, which is typical of so many responses to the book.

CASE HISTORY 1—NIGHT WAKING, JOINT PAIN

—based on records kept from birth. This is to illustrate the problems caused in healthy breast-fed children who may never suffer obvious major allergic disease.

Philip, our first child, was born in February 1976. Pregnancy had been uneventful except for considerable heartburn, for which I drank *more* milk. I was fully breast-fed for 9 months, and have had only minor inhalant allergies, though bottle-fed relations suffer from asthma. Philip's father, Jim, was largely bottle-fed after rigid scheduled breast-feeding failed; had bronchitis and other problems throughout childhood, but was 'well' until a serious bout of gastroenteritis in adulthood. He has since realized that many 'minor' health problems are caused by his multiple food sensitivities, especially milk.

Philip's birth was traumatic—prolonged labour, many drugs, eventually Keilland's forceps delivery. Although big and healthy, Philip was therefore kept in a special nursery for 36 hours. I became engorged and in rapid succession developed all the breast and nipple problems possible, largely as a result of poor management. Regular complementary feeds of formula, no night feeding, scheduled day feeds, etc. all guaranteed a low and decreasing supply of milk. Therefore I was given gallons of milk heavily fortified with skim milk powder and chocolate (in the quite erroneous belief that extra fluid and protein rather than extra suckling would increase my supply).

Philip was reasonably content for the first few weeks. As with many babies, severe colic did not begin until 3 weeks, and did not end—tho' it improved—around 3 months. Against much well-meant advice, we continued to believe that he was in pain, as he seemed to be. (We tried drugs and everything else, but nothing worked—he lived in a sling most of the time, as he seemed more comfortable there than lying down.)

Food for thought

Eventually, the intensity of the pain seemed to diminish, turning into extreme night restlessness and waking in pain. I continued to breast-feed him, and took him into bed with us, as this was the only way we got enough sleep to cope. As soon as he was able to speak, he complained of stomach and leg pains—diagnosed as 'growing pains'. He was exclusively breast-fed till $4\frac{1}{2}$ months, and partly for over three years. (His earliest weaning foods included yoghurt, banana, honey, cheese—all foods he can't tolerate now.)

Christmas day 1979 we were out for lunch, and the kids gorged on sweets, ice cream, crisps, soft drinks. That night Philip was hospitalized with intense abdominal pain. Healthy appendix removed, he then suffered repeated bowel obstructions losing 30 per cent of his body weight over a period of days on an intravenous drip. His convalescent diet was cows' milk (chocolate flavoured) and orange and pineapple juices. Probable lactose intolerance developed—he had stools so fluid and acid that they blistered the whole of his back—but no tests were done, and my concern about diet was ignored. In the end I substituted fresh expressed breast milk, and he stopped having spasms of gut pain, and no further obstruction developed. The surgeon stated that Philip's pain was due to mesenteric adenitis, and he was surprised that it proved to be so persistent. I have since learnt of numerous other cases of mesentenic adenitis which were related to foods, not viruses.

Because of the diarrhoea, Philip was given no cows' milk as such during his convalescence at home. (By now I had realized that he had been milk-intolerant as a baby, but believed that he had 'grown out of it', as it is dogmatically asserted that children do.) However, he had milk in other forms, and his night waking and joint pains continued till August 1980, when I read an article linking joint disease and food intolerance. A trial elimination of milk resulted in sleep so peaceful that we thought he'd died! Any night waking from then on could always be traced to milk in some form—and even though he loved it, Philip willingly gave it up.

In late December 1980, Philip ate a Jatz cracker with $\frac{1}{4}$ in cube of cheese. That night he had pain as severe as mesenteric adenitis of Christmas 1979. The next night he had severe croup and wheeze, with no aftermath next day—no obvious infection. We tested this a month later, with the same result. In February 1981 he began school and woke in pain every second night for 2 weeks. On pain days, Philip took bread for lunch, so we investigated. Local baker admitted 'throwing in a handful' of skim milk in each batch. Baker stopped this; night pain stopped. (How easily this could have been diagnosed as trouble adjusting to school!)

Over 1981 other sensitivities were recognized: citrus fruits, preservatives, artificial colours and flavours,? grapes,? some stone fruits, beef. These cause less severe symptoms, although headache, temperature rise, nose bleeds, and earache are now symptoms, and his rhinitis is more severe. Inhalants are now also involved, especially petrochemicals and house dust. As he can articulate what he feels, he is an excellent observer, and has very seldom tried to 'use' his disability. In the few doubtful cases, when he's trying to get out of school, for example, there are objective

Case histories

measures such as pulse and temperature, stools and appetite, to check. On the whole, he is completely reliable and not prone to exaggeration—if he says he is having a reaction, he is. He is aware of subtle changes in his body. This enables early symptomatic treatment, which seems to lessen the severity of the attack and the likelihood of secondary infection. And being taken seriously and treated appropriately seems to have prevented any behavioural effects: he gets sympathy in a very matter of fact way, and does not get angry that no-one believes him, or grumpy because he doesn't feel right inside and everyone thinks he's 'putting on'.

In 1982, penicillin administered when Philip was having a mild reaction, and when in hindsight he probably had threadworms, resulted in a major reaction: blotches all over his body. (He had had penicillin before over the years, with no problems.) Chemical sensitivities at school also became a bother. His frequent night nose bleeds, stopped when we removed his dacron pillow—subsequent allergy testing indicated sensitivity to dacron. (He has a wool pillow in a cotton case.)

As a baby, he also had snuffles off and on, dreadful hiccoughs, peculiar breathing at times, persistent cradle cap (which finally disappeared when milk eliminated), frequent possetting, excessive wind. While still fully breast-fed he had a few 'colds', once solids were introduced these began as cough, with runny eyes and nose.

Philip has sisters, 24 and 21 months apart. Neither was given anything but breast milk for their first 5 months of life; neither had one of the symptoms above. Both were placid, cheerful, 'model' babies who only cried when hungry, cold, tired, or bored. Maternal diet in pregnancy and lactation had not altered significantly; believing that 'comps' were the significant factor for Philip, I still had around two litres of milk each day. I was significantly more tired and had more difficulties with each pregnancy. Both siblings' births were induced; the third labour was precipitate and the child's breathing depressed due to overuse of oxytocin and unasked-for pethidine just before delivery. Third child's Apgar score was lowest, and the post-partum period most difficult, of the three children. That child, Elizabeth, had consistently refused to drink more than a mouthful of cows' milk until about three years old. Lately she had begun to have small quantities of milk and yoghurt, but if she eats more than about $\frac{1}{2}$ oz of cheese, she has an extremely restless night, arm pains, and loose stools. The middle child, Katie, flourished while breast-fed (until 15 months) but has had growth problems since around 2 years old—on a normal diet including plenty of milk. We are still working on that problem! [Postscript 1984: Katie too is milk-sensitive. She was, we discover from the hospital records, given two 20 ml feeds of Lactogen within 6 hours of birth—contrary to hospital policy, our doctor's and our written instructions and the notes on her cot.]

All three children are healthy, bright, and have no behavioural problems. They are rarely sick—though Elizabeth at 23 months had a bout of diarrhoea which lasted a week. During that time she reverted to full breast-feeding and fluids and ORS supplementation (cf. p. 135); she was perfectly cheerful and alert throughout. (Shortly after this our local doc-

Food for thought

tor's daughter caught the same bug, was given lucozade *et al.* and ended up in hospital on an intravenous drip for 5 days.) Philip can now cope with small quantities of some former allergens but must still avoid milk absolutely, which we've all adjusted to.

Many similar 'minor' cases where colic is succeeded by night restlessness, joint pains, and other 'normal' problems have since been reported. This is probably a fairly typical subclinical case, where the medical problems were relatively minor (to all but the child experiencing the pain), but the family would be very different, had the parents not identified the physical cause of a very physical problem. The label given to a problem can be part of the solution or part of a greater problem, as the second case history may illustrate.

CASE HISTORY 2— BEHAVIOURAL EFFECTS

—In this case, the consequences for the child and his family were far worse. Marital breakdown was the result of family tension over mother's 'inadequate' handling of the child; mother's self-esteem has been badly damaged. Child's life has been a nightmare.

Jonathon (not his real name)
Born 1973
Birth Bottle-fed—Lactogen, later switched to cows' milk. Bad wind, colic, cried a lot. Crawled at 8 months, but not for long, and in unusual manner; could not take out because he was always angry. Rocked and cried.
12 months. Walked. Easily, frustrated; breaks everything; impatient; always crying; throws things; tantrums; always hungry, continuous bottles; eats and throws food everywhere, sticks it in ears; doesn't sleep for long, up all night, into sugar, flour tea. Gets into things, attention seeking. Sore throats, earaches.
18 months. Broke cot, so into bed; bangs head on wall, punches door and walls; rips curtains, bedspread, and sheets; takes off soiled nappies, smears walls, fills cracks with faeces and cakes nose and ears with same.
2 years. Puts fist through window; hyperactive; in car tries to climb out of window, pulls on handbrake, and tries to open door of moving car; first noticed very sensitive skin, screamed when dressed in nylon clothes, lying on grass brought him out in German-measle-type blotches; had sunburn after short exposure; sore throat, earaches.
3 years. Temper getting worse, running away, tries to drown cat. Headaches, earaches.
4 years. Broke a glass divider in bathroom in fit of temper (using hammer). Noticed very bad body odour.
5 years. At infant school has trouble discriminating colours, used black almost exclusively. Hates school, comes home in temper fit, difficulty in getting him to school next day. Unco-operative, fights, bad temper. Always thirsty, aches in all joints; tonsils and adenoids removed.

Case histories

6 years. Smacking useless, fights back; throws table and chairs; cries before and after school. Depressed, won't come out of room, smashes car window in temper, hates mother and sister; thinks former became ill to hurt him. Headaches, pains in joints; dreams see faces and eyes, becomes very frightened by this. Ear operation.

7 years. Continuation of above; refuses to sleep without light on.

8 years. Wants to kill mother and sister with knife and cricket bat; necessary to hide all sharp implements, likely weapons; uncontrollable; counselling from community health service—of little value.

9 years! 'Feels different'; temper worse; punches, kicks; breaks couch in fit; won't go to bed till 11–12 at night; cannot reason with him; rides off on bike and doesn't come home; gets up on house roof and will not come down. Demands attentions, wants mother to play with him all the time; tries an experiment in pantry and nearly sets fire to place, indicating an inability to judge appropriateness of, and consequence of his actions. Scared to sleep without light on at night; despite heat, sleeps with bedroom door shut, but with fan on, likes the vibrations. Sleep walks. Depression, tension, fatigue, can't be rushed, has never dressed himself; rolls around floor when putting on T-shirts. Will not eat at regular mealtimes, picky with food, eats all day, junk food, drinks 2–3 litres of milk a day, has food fads, gained 2 stone in weight in 7 months. Always had bad cradle cap, now has dandruff; itchiness, sweatiness; easy bruising, irritability, rashes from contact/exposure to wool, nylon, grass, sun. Rings under eyes; frequent colds, night cough, stomach pains. Rubs eyes, complains of something in them, sits 6 inches from television, has visual distortions when riding in car. Family counselling from psychologist of no benefit to family or Jonathon.

Comments

Work commenced with Jonathon 3rd term 1980. At that time he could not read or write, lacked numeracy skills; his ability to learn was hampered by lack of concentration, short attention span and defective audioverbal memory. His co-operation as far as his ability to attend would allow was good. However his behaviour at home was still no better and progress in the learning sphere was extremely slow. He was tried on diet in 1981 together with supplementary B3 and Compound Zinc. At this time he was drinking 2–3 litres of milk. There was no significant, long term change in behaviour.

March 1982 a strict elimination diet was started in an endeavour to determine the presence of food allergies. Carrots, beans, peas send him right off. He does get extremely irritable when his mother and sister eat foods which he is not allowed. There seems to be a distinct possibility that cigarette smoke triggers an outburst of irrational behaviour.

About the time Jonathon commenced the new eating regime a different approach to the development of short memory, and to teaching speech sound discrimination was begun. The improvement has been dramatic. Jonathon is now capable of retaining a complex sequence for the time

Food for thought

required to successfully complete the activity. He has begun reading voluntarily, and although (as can be expected) needs help, he is reading independently for the first time in his life. These changes confirm a belief I have held for some time, that is, in a significant number of children the disturbed functioning of the metabolism must be corrected *before* any real progress can occur either in the behavioural or learning sphere.

The foregoing was written by the teacher was has been working with Jonathon, Ruth Millar.

In this type of problem child, years of learned behaviour won't be undone by the diet. The family's expectations of, and responses to, Jonathon have not been magically altered. Their behaviour, and his, will take a lot of time and patience to change. Support for such families is critical, as other addicts have learnt—witness AA and Al-Anon. It is also highly probable that his mother's behaviour is influenced by food and chemical addictants, and she has not yet been able to tackle this problem (not surprisingly!).

However, when an elimination diet was first suggested, no one imagined that Jonathon would have the comprehension and will power to give up his favourite foods. (He threw tantrums over being restricted.) The fact that he has persevered, has improved so much, and feels so much better that he keeps to the diet, is testimony to how great a role these simple things can play even in extreme cases. A neurologist who works with Vietnam veterans says this child's behaviour is amazingly like that of the veterans. Had the diet failed, he would have tried to work with Jonathon. (There is no place in Victoria where *child* addicts, unable to keep to a diet, may be hospitalized and fasted as adults are.)

CASE HISTORY 3—ECZEMA

—Boy, $2\frac{1}{2}$, 'comp'-fed in hospital, breast-fed thereafter.

From about 6 weeks old he had little dry patches of skin on his eyebrows and forehead but other than that was perfectly healthy and happy baby until about 9 months . . . when I put him on the bottle (cows' milk) he reacted violently . . . He lost a lot of weight and his skin became really bad . . . He was just a mess, and became very unhappy. The doctor diagnosed eczema. I took him to a paediatrician who prescribed creams which didn't help . . . His hands would react to different foods as he fed himself. In trying to find out all the foods he was allergic to I nearly starved him. I tried to get a doctor's assistance but they just said idiotic things like—'he'll grow out of it'.

Well, I have watched him suffer now for 2 years and a placid happy baby has become a very miserable, bad tempered, angry little boy. He has hands and feet like those of an old man which I bandage every day so that he doesn't tear the flesh of them.

Case histories

Since going to a GP who investigated diet, this child is almost totally symptom-free. A similar case was publicized in a national women's magazine—a child of 4 who had been bandaged from head to toe every day for years; monthly chemist's bills of £25. Her parents know now what foods cause a flare-up; she is bandage-free.

CASE HISTORY 4—ASTHMA AND BRONCHIAL COMPLAINTS

—Boy, 9, 'comp'-fed in hospital, breast-fed afterwards. Severe colic; weaned at 3 months, 4 months, eczema appeared, continued until 2 years old; controlled by steroid creams.

Baby was now consuming great amounts of his beloved cows' milk. At $2\frac{1}{2}$ years he suddenly became asthmatic. Paediatrician consulted and our child classified as an allergic type who would improve with age. Winters of bronchitis, pneumonia, and many asthma episodes followed.

At the time I was working part time in a nursery of approximately 40 babies under 2, at least five were medically proven allergic to cows' milk. These babies were constantly suffering respiratory illness and were grossly overweight. I cut back on milk in family diet but did not eliminate all dairy products.

Fortunately, I happened to attend a GP who, because of his own asthma, has a great interest in allergies . . .

. . . Proper investigations revealed multiple food and inhalant intolerances. 'It is more than likely that the scene was set by the cows' milk allergy . . . I feel great frustration when I think of the damage done by my own and the medical profession's ignorance.

The child's asthma is now well controlled by dietary means. This boy's sister was 2 weeks premature and 'comp-fed' . . .

Well-meaning hospital staff were pushing jugs of cows' milk at me and I, equally ignorant, obligingly consumed same. After 6 weeks I almost weaned, having a baby full of colic. Thanks to my doctor, I didn't—he handed me a tin of Prosobee and literature about cows' milk intolerance as a cause of colic. The colic disappeared as if by magic.

A third child, weeks premature, and very ill, was fed EBM (expressed breast milk) exclusively. There were no signs of allergy until . . .

about a month after commencing solids I noticed some dry patches appearing on his legs. Over a period of 6 months these became more

181

Food for thought

eczema-like . . . I showed the rash to my other son's specialist and he suggested eliminating dairy products. In 5 days his skin was clear. Two weeks later I tested by reintroducing dairy products and in 48 hours the rash returned. I will test once more but I feel the evidence is conclusive.

This mother ended by saying

Even though I feel my third child is probably equally as sensitive as the first, with a totally different approach and diet we have an entirely different result. I feel for my elder son, who has had to suffer 6 years of asthma needlessly!

CASE HISTORY 5— RECURRENT PROBLEMS; INFANT DIARRHOEA

Mother breast-feeding a colicky, slow-gaining baby eliminated dairy products from the family diet (to save doing two lots of cooking). Colicky baby stopped screaming and his diarrhoea improved. His older siblings, aged 8 and 6, amazed the specialist who had been treating them for recurrent tonsillitis and otitis media—scheduled operations were cancelled. That spring the family did not suffer from, their usual hayfever, older children remained free of colds and ear infections. Baby now medically diagnosed cows' milk intolerant. At 19 months given milk with morning cereal for 4 days, then Combantrim for worms. Acute diarrhoeal episode followed, very badly managed for 4 days (no breast milk, flat lemonade etc.). Within 24 hours of reverting to breast-feeding and giving ORS solution, child was 'as good as gold'. Any subsequent diarrhoea managed with ORS and breast—child never at risk. (Had been hospitalized more than once during previous bouts.) Parents amazed and angry that no-one had ever told them what to do for infant diarrhoea.

CASE HISTORY 6 — TODDLER DIARRHOEA

To summarize this file, which extended over months, is very difficult:

Boy of 2½ had chronic bulky loose stools, rapid weight fluctuation, allergic rhinitis, recurrent colds, ear infections, etc. Frequent bouts of diarrhoea, with consequent endless washing and cleaning to be done; no hope of toilet training. Mother reached the point where she almost felt that she couldn't bear to touch another dirty nappy, or even the child, without losing control. Not until the child born 9 lb + was under the 10th percentile was this considered to be a 'medical' problem—mother received clear messages about her neurosis, obsessiveness being the 'real' problem. After home testing, parents sure that milk was part of the problem. Doctor suggested 2 week trial of 1 oz dairy products daily. Over the first week child lost 8 oz and parents were 'reduced to throwing a bucket of water and disinfectant over him and the front steps.' Doctor still not con-

Case histories

vinced—tried Flagyl because giardia might perhaps be the problem. Severe reaction: rhinitis, bronchitis, contact rash around mouth, diarrhoea. Doctor finally convinced—several drugs prescribed and parents followed diet they had worked out by themselves. At three, child was '100 per cent better than before the diet and drugs', although asthma had emerged and nose and gut symptoms were present in mild forms. Friends found it difficult to recognize the child. Four months later, in spring and after a vacation away from home, child had severe diarrhoeal relapse. Subsided after 10 days—child never seriously ill:
   This child's symptoms are reasonably well controlled and the family is happy with the accommodation they have reached. In their particular circumstances, thorough diagnosis and treatment is impossible, so the child is unlikely to be symptom-free for lengthy periods.

SUMMARY

None of these children had only one symptom, or only one problem food or inhalant. In no case were there behavioural effects without other physical effects as well, although I am sometimes misrepresented as suggesting this. It was necessary to omit all the minor details that mothers reported so ably; and I also omitted the more trenchant comments made, particularly by those mothers whose children had suffered appallingly for years. I did not recount such cases, but only a sample of fairly representative, medically 'not serious' cases. But I feel other mothers should have the last word:

I wish the medical profession was more informed on the subject, especially on the side they do not see in hospitals—i.e., problems that are too small to see a doctor over ... The nurses kept saying 'That is most unusual' in a tone that implied that I didn't know what I was talking about. Yet you know, and I know, that none of this is at all unusual.

And from a doctor mother:

Your radio talks came at a time when I was struggling with a colicky, rashy breast-fed baby and no single thing in my diet seemed to be the cause. Your findings gave me sufficient moral support to persist and eventually milk/eggs/tomatoes/pineapple/apricot/carrot? proved culprits. Life improved dramatically.
   I found it all doubly difficult to cope with as being a trained doctor I (a) was expected to know about colic by infant health clinics etc. (I didn't) (b) was discouraged by lack of information in medical literature (felt if it was all true, somebody would definitely have proved it by now.) So many thanks again.

23

Food intolerance and food aversion: a joint report by the Royal College of Physicians and the British Nutrition Foundation

CONCLUSIONS AND CRITICISMS

This is a major report, and must be carefully read by all those interested in the subject. Its conclusions, here reproduced with permission, do not convey enough of what the Report contains. But they emphasize both the complexity of the problems parents currently face and the need to work co-operatively with orthodox medical practitioners, if at all possible.

CONCLUSIONS

1. Reactions of food intolerance have gained increasing recognition in recent years but the lack of adequate scientifically based research and the lack of medical interest has led to the proliferation of organisations, centres and individuals offering advice and which has little scientific basis.
2. A wide variety of symptoms have been incorrectly attributed to the effects of foods; even when the attribution is correct, there has been confusion between conditions caused by allergy, enzyme deficiencies, pharmacological reactions, psychological reactions and other mechanisms. Food intolerance can both mimic other conditions and be mimicked by them.
3. No estimate can be made of the prevalence of food intolerance because of a lack of adequate information. With the exception of rare but specific biochemical defects, diagnostic methods still depend on dietary studies or on a psychiatric assessment and are highly subjective.
4. The dietary approach to the management of food intolerance is particularly complex and may lead to nutritional difficulties and social disruption. There are considerable dangers in the unsupervised use of diets, especially for infants and young children.
5. For those patients who react abnormally to components of various foods, there is a need for better access to information on the ingredients of foods beyond what is given on the label.
6. Emotional difficulties are common and may sometimes be secondary to immunological or other types of food reaction. Whatever the aetiology, these patients are often ill and in need of treatment which takes account of

their psychological and emotional needs as well as any physical aspects of their food intolerance.

Criticisms

To incorporate references to this recently published Report in this book has meant going back through the text after copy-editing, something every editor and author would prefer not to do. But I see the Report as providing substantial support for much that was written in 1982/3 and was then regarded as somewhat radical. Most of my textural references made it clear that I am delighted with the report. For such a group to write like this must do a great deal to persuade the sceptics, lay and medical, that food intolerance will not go away as a problem, so they had better read more on the subject. (Here too the Report is useful, as a starting-point for those who want references.)

However, certain aspects of the Report deserve criticism. I have already noted the weakness of the discussion on infant colic and maternal diet. Overall, the least scientific section was that on the psychological aspects of food intolerance.[1] Here there is much that is unexceptional—social pressures undoubtedly contribute to eating disorders, whether in women or men. (It would have been good for such a Report to suggest ways of reducing such pressures by controls on advertising targeted at vulnerable groups, education of consumers, etc.) The underlying message of this section however, is that psychosomatic mechanisms account for a great deal of this present vogue of food intolerance and that women are anxious, insecure, and neurotic creatures who produce these problems in their children. Psychological food intolerance can be distinguished from physiological food intolerance by the 'failure to reproduce an adverse reaction when the patient is unaware that the food has been consumed, i.e., when it has been administered by a naso-gastric tube'.[2] The Report claims that patients who refuse to accept such a diagnosis can be shown to be more likely to be psychiatrically disordered.

This will be familiar to many readers as the sort of 'help' they have been offered every many years before they discovered the true causes of their problems. On what does it rest? Two studies are basic. One, of just 23 patients,[3] is implicitly criticized on p. 18 of the Report itself because 'relatively small quantities of food in capsules may be sufficient to trigger allergic reactions but . . .

185

larger amounts may be necessary to provoke other types of food intolerance.' The study failed to provoke reactions in 19 patients using this now dubious method. Indeed, since the Egger findings on migraine,[4] I would have hoped that all researchers realized the difficulty of relying on any standardized procedure such as this! The second study showed that those with irritable bowel syndrome showed 'a significantly greater improvement when psychotherapy was part of the treatment.[5] This is not in conflict with the possibility of physiological food intolerance—various therapies can improve the body's ability to cope with food problems, from massage, exercise, and relaxation techniques to psychotherapy. An improvement therefore says nothing about the basic etiology of the problem. Psychological stress occurs in real bodies, and may involve the liberation of many chemical mediators which could potentiate food responses. Teaching patients how to manage stress can be expected to improve symptoms in those for whom stress is a problem. And being taken seriously, allowed to talk to someone who listens, is a powerful therapy in people used to being dismissed as hypochondriacs. Conversely, NOT being taken seriously, observing your doctor conclude that you are another neurotic female, or an 'old woman' (revealing phrase) has a detrimental effect on the mental health of the sanest of us.[6] It creates anxiety, self-doubt, and stress. After years of such treatment from various doctors, it would be remarkable if patients with undiagnosed illness were not more prone to psychiatric disorders. Being hostile to psychiatric diagnosis[7] can be the right and proper response for those many people who retain some measure of confidence in their own knowledge of their minds and bodies. How many times does medicine have to be mistaken before doctors learn to stop ascribing to psychological *causes* all and any symptoms for which they currently have no physiological explanation?

Does the patient's absence of symptoms when unaware of challenge constitute psychological intolerance? Possibly, in rare cases. Probably not, in many. Naso-gastric tubes are criticized in the Report[8] itself, as by-passing areas where attacks may be triggered—in some people the oral mucosa and oesophagus can be important sites for antigen response. But even if one could administer the same dose in the same way and the same combination of feeds, without the patient knowing, the knowledge itself (and the fear response it brings in people who have had repeated adverse effects) may be simply a potentiating factor, akin to exercise in food-dependent exercise-induced anaphylaxis.

As for food intolerance by proxy[9] (cf. p. 66)—families are often right when they refuse to accept their child's behaviour as appropriate considering their circumstances. Precarious family equilibrium can be the result of quarrels over the affected child—the mother senses strongly that the child is not responsible for the problem, the father blames his wife as unable to manage the child, the child becomes the focus of family resentment.[10] The role of the doctor is often to exacerbate the tensions by psychological diagnoses and drug prescription. Subject any adults to prolonged sleep deprivation, then tell them that it is really their doing, that all they have to do is to manage an inexplicably distressed and non-verbal person better . . . As a recipe for mental disorders this would be hard to beat. The description[11] of these families sounds to me like many Australian food-intolerant families with a history of allergy, intelligent (not 'pre-morbid'—how could that be defined?) and united concern, and a willingness to explore any avenue that offers hope (is that 'gullible'?). The interesting thing is that these Australian families had spent their 'large sums of money' not on alternative but on orthodox medicine, without ever being convinced of a word their expensive consultants said when experience proved them wrong.[12] Because they persisted, they were all properly diagnosed in the end, and their health immeasurably improved. Eating disorders such as anorexia and bulimia are also discussed. If I were a bookmaker, I would not accept any bets that in 20 years' time medicine will not have uncovered more substantial links between these disorders and true food intolerance, aversion, and addiction alike, though at present I accept social and cultural explanations.

Other criticisms of the Report concern the implicit definition of healthy people (apparently those who do not consult doctors about ailments are suitable 'healthy' controls for those who do!)[13] and of normal childhood health.[14] What guarantees have we that the *usual* childhood symptoms do not reflect the usual pattern of childhood food-intolerant responses? (see p. 33).

There is also little basis for the Report's certainty that the incidence of food allergy (or other intolerances) is greatest in the first few months of life and decreases with age,[15] in either the Australian experience or a remarkable Finnish report—also overlooked—which showed that the incidence actually increased between one and three years of age (19 per cent to 27 per cent), dropping back to 8 per cent by the age of six.[16] It would be interesting to follow those children through life, particularly into pregnancy and beyond.

Another omission was a thorough discussion of the prophylactic value of *exclusive* breast-feeding from birth until 6 months. Until very recently the importance of detailed records of infant diet was not fully appreciated (see p. 15). Two separate centres have recently reported substantial differences in allergy when exclusively breast-fed infants are investigated; one showed clearly that when babies are exclusively breast-fed, rates of allergy are lower when other foods are introduced after 6 months.[17] (As compared with those receiving other foods after 3 to 5 months.) But perhaps these studies were published too late to influence this Report, although earlier[18] work by some of the same authors was not noted either.

Nor is there any discussion about possible links between childhood food intolerance (which is 'grown out of') and adult food reactions. Yet we are told on p. 17 of the Report that even strict food allergy (probably the least common of intolerant reactions) 'is by no means rare'. Is this *de novo* adult intolerance, or are we looking at these same children who 'grew out of it'? Or both? For instance, joint pains, and the ability of foods to exacerbate inflammatory joint disease in adults, is discussed, albeit cautiously;[19] yet joint pains in childhood, frequently 'diagnosed' as 'growing pains', are nowhere mentioned in the Report. This is one of the most common minor manifestations of food intolerance in the families on whom my work has been based. Similarly, 'abdomenal migraine' is a common descriptive diagnosis for symptoms of abdominal pain, sometimes with loose stools. This could be primary sucrase-isomaltase deficiency, discussed on p. 25 of the Report, or it could be mesenteric adenitis, as it was in my son's case (see p. 175). In either case it is indeed likely to be 'misconstrued as a reflection of maternal anxiety.'[20] This is an acknowledgement from the report that we mothers may sometimes be right and be put off with psychological nonsense.

However throughout the Report we 'patients' (we are becoming much less patient nowadays!) are either entirely passive, mistaken, misguided, obsessive, neurotic, or otherwise difficult. When

Food intolerance and food aversion

we do something right, it is not the result of careful observation of our child and its behaviour; rather, 'mothers may unconsciously select a low protein diet'[21] in cases where symptoms are made worse by protein. At no stage is there any conception of the intolerant person as an active participant in the process of diagnosis or decision-making about testing or management—yet it is very clear to me that if people are not individually educated, motivated, and convinced, compliance in every area will be poor and the results disappointing.

Is the solution then, to use dietary manipulation only as a last resort and rely heavily on 'relatively simple and efficacious' drugs?[22] I have discussed this in earlier sections of this book. Here I should like to record my disappointment that the Report did not adopt a more critical approach to the use of drugs. None are entirely free of hazards, and the allergic/intolerant patient is more at risk than others. That there is as yet little evidence of common adverse effects may be a result of such uncritical acceptance. Drugs for the intolerant patient have included preservatives, colourings, and flavourings all known to cause reactions that in some patients can be life-threatning. Using lactose as the vehicle to administer on inhalant drug for example, has to carry some risk that the lactose is contaminated with milk protein to which the person may react violently. Australia uses more broncho-dilators than any other country; its dairy industry has been heavily promoting milk to the teenage/young adult market; and the asthma death rate continues to rise yearly. Are there any connections between these facts? Assuming drugs to be safe will not help uncover them if they aren't. Perhaps another explanation for the observed fact that tartrazine reactions are reportedly more common for pharmaceutical preparations than for food and drink[23] is that the drug component in some way potentiates the reactions, where certain foods ameliorate it. Again, this is speculative, but presuming drugs to be safe will prevent any such interactions from being easily observed.

Of course, any such Report represents an attempt to summarize a very difficult problem, and to represent that which is currently accepted by leading practitioners. The views and practices of such people can vary, according to their assumptions and experience. (we all have assumptions that are useful or harmful in particular cases: mine, that parents generally can be trusted not to want extra

189

problems, and to know their children, arises from my experience of caring intelligent parents. I recognize in theory that all sorts of other parents exist, but do not instinctively assume that parents are anxious, obsessive creatures who create their problems out of their psychological needs. Doctors who *have* met such parents must be affected by it. Where I might fail to recognize one such, they might mistakenly classify a caring parent as neurotic.) There *are* minor divergences in the Report that suggest different approaches and assumptions were blended in the final product. All such documents are a state-of-the-art summary, and as such are to some extent out of date before they are printed. None the less they serve a useful purpose—so long as they are not treated as the final word by those who find in them material to support their views. Too often official reports are used as cudgels to suppress currently unproven theories. Their great value is that they usually contain material acceptable to all sides in any debate. I can see this Report being quoted with relish not only by me, but also by those who see food intolerance as rare, the latest fad of neurotic middle-class mothers, and so on. This would all be good clean fun if only parents were able to talk back on equal terms and if we had access to medical channels of communication and debate. For we argue from a position of weakness. We have no say in funding, there are no channels for us to put our case to doctors. When bizarre cases[24] are uncovered and reported as showing the harm done by self-diagnosis, or lay help, we cannot reply showing equally devastating cases due to medical misdiagnosis and mismanagement—not because they do not exist, but because no one wants to know about such cases. (For doctors to openly begin acknowledging mistakes, or criticizing one another's practices, would inevitably lead to more, and more successful, lawsuits. Unless, of course, patients were truly educated, so that they understood the reasons behind a doctor's decisions, realized that he is a fallible, hard-working individual and that genuine mistakes are inevitable.)

Without more and better communication, the two groups will continue to diverge, to their mutual loss. This book is my attempt to bridge that gap.

24

Resources

This is not intended as a complete list of relevant resources. Some of the books listed in the further reading section contain useful directories, and there is no point in duplicating their work. If you write to small self-help groups, do enclose stamps: it all mounts up, and most have very little money.

1. THE PRIMARY RESOURCE: YOU

To achieve any real change there is a need for interested groups to develop a network system which minimizes duplication of effort and maximizes the spread of knowledge about our common problems. This is developing rapidly in Australia, where the Allergy Association has mushroomed into every state, and the Australian Consumers' Association has agreed to act as a clearing house for information. There is no room for approaches which divide patients according to their symptoms—asthma, eczema, hyperactivity, whatever—when some of the major underlying causes may be identical. Such groups certainly have their uses, but they need to co-operate with others on issues of common concern, such as food and drug labelling, infant feeding practices, etc. For example, one group could press for a radical update of knowledge about what percentage of drugs and chemicals given to mothers are ingested by their breast-feeding infants, since current figures seem to be based often on single-figure numbers of women studied. Other groups might produce lists of practitioners, clinics, and local contacts who can be relied upon to give support when families are going through food-intolerance crises. Knowing that you can ring a sympathetic listener can be a great help. Gaining knowledge about your illness and being more able to make your own decisions about treatment is a real confidence-builder and a valuable part of getting better. Unfortunately, too many people are simply looking for ways to put the responsibility for their health on to doctors. We allow, or even invite, the professionals to tell us how we should be treated and remain passive and unquestioning in the seemingly

Food for thought

endless diagnostic journey from GP to hospital, to out-patients', to clinic, back to GP and despair, picking up drugs, inconclusive diagnoses, prognoses, and labels along the way. This does not make for good medicine, nor for good health—mental or physical. We accept the blame for being sick, but not the responsibility of getting well, and of finding ways of controlling those social problems which help to make us ill. We don't talk to doctors, telling them what has helped and what has not—yet we blame them for not realizing how useless the treatment was.

Of course, as a patient and non-doctor, I understand why we don't, and doctors' attitudes and lifestyles are part of the answer. But we can only change ourselves, and then hope that our doctor will have the ability to change with us. Blaming them for being the product of their education is pointless and counterproductive. Rather, rejoice in the fact that so many remain interested, concerned human beings despite their workload! And concentrate on becoming involved with them, even in the medical decision-making process.

But keeping in touch with similar groups should not mean giving up other contacts. Childbirth and parenting groups, civic and service clubs, even senior citizens' groups, all have common interests with 'allergy'. Helping them to see this makes life easier all around—'allergy' is not some minority crankiness but a major community problem. Community education, and broadly based support, will be an essential part of any strategy for change.

It is not possible to give a detailed account of the situation in every country. But there are plenty of local experts, and resources, and publications for you to follow up. Get involved, now, if you are concerned about this subject. Ask questions of manufacturers, and pass on your learning. Nothing will happen if everyone leaves it to the next person to do it all.

2. UK RESOURCES

(A) Directories

A few directories of health resources which overlap with topics covered in this book are in print or in preparation. To locate them or to have your own group included, they are as follows:

College of Health, 18 Victoria Park Square, London E2 9PS.

Resources

Aim to provide a consumer association for patients and to place patients and practitioners on more equal terms. The College has an index of Self-health Groups and is planning to provide them with an information service. They also publish a quarterly journal *Self health*.

Share Community Limited, Alexandra House, 140 Battersea Park Road, London SW11 4NB. Tel: 01–622–6885.
Share community assist mentally and physically disabled people. They run a self-help information bank and publish *Guide to self-help groups*.

National Council for Voluntary Organizations (NCVO), 26 Bedford Square. London WC1B 3HV. Tel: 01–636–4066.
Assist voluntary organizations at all levels. If, for example, you aimed to set up local groups providing support and/or health care for food-intolerance sufferers, NCVO have a Community Health Initiatives Resource Unit which you could Contact at the above address.

Ruth West and Joanna Trevelyan, KIB Foundation, 23 Harley House, Marylebone Road, London NW1 5H. Tel: 01–487–4261.
They are producing a bibliography on alternative medicine. They're tracking down 3000 references covering major areas in the field.

See also Thames Television in the Bibliography. (p. 213).

(B) Allergy and the environment: resource groups/contacts

Unfortunately I cannot judge the competence or otherwise of all of these listed, as I have had no personal or secondhand experience of some. Don't presume that all that you read is gospel truth—*caveat emptor*! I would welcome feedback from UK readers who do contact any of these and try out their ideas.

Action Against Allergy (Mrs Amelia Nathan-Hill), 43 The Downs, London SW20 8GH. Tel: 01–540–2273.
Mrs Hill has a bookshop at 31 Abbey Parade, Merton High St, London SW19 1DG, which can supply most books on this subject.

Action on Smoking & Health, Margaret Pyke House, 27–35 Mortimer St., London W1N 7RJ. Tel: 01–637–9843.

Allergy Advisory Service, Mrs W.E. Simmonds, SRN, 20 Taunton Road, Pedwell, Bridgewater, Somerset TA7 9BG.

Food for thought

Information, advice about elimination and rotation diets. Can supply detailed information on diets for home use. Send £1.50 and a large SAE.

Appropriate Health Resources & Technologies Action Group (AHRTAG), 85 Marylebone High Street, London W1M 3DE.

Association for Optimum Nutrition, Upper Vicars Farm, Stonechurch, Bucks HP14 3YL.

Promote vitamin therapy, and publish a directory of nutritional practitioners and organizations.

Asthma Society and Friends of the Asthma Research Council, 12 Pembridge Square, London W2 4EH. Tel: 01–229–1142.

Local branches; help and information.

Barbara Dickinson, 7 Manor Road, Duckington, Oxford OX8 7YD.

Runs a postal group who offer help with baby problems, colic, sleep disturbances, food allergy, hyperactivity, eczma, and sickly baby syndrome. She specializes in help with babies with food allergy. SAE (large) required.

British Migraine Association, 178A High Road, Byfleet, Weybridge, Surrey KT14 7ED. Tel: 09323–52468.

Campaign for Lead-Free Air (CLEAR), 2 North Down Street London N1 9BG.

Chemical Victims, 12 Highlands Road, Worting, Near Basingstoke, Hants.

Childrens' Help Line, (Basingstoke), Ocean View, Bishopswood Lane, Baughurst, Hants. Tel: Tadley 6662.

Coeliac Society of the UK. P.O. Box 181, London NW2 2QY.

Consumers Association, Buckingham Street, London WC2N 6DS. Tel: 01–839–1222.

Drugs Information and Advisory Service, 111 Cowbridge Rd. East Cardiff CF19 AG. Tel: 0222–26113 (24 hrs).

SAE for publications list.

Food and Chemical Allergy Association, (Chairman, Mrs E. Rothera), 27 Ferringham Lane, Ferring-by-Sea, West Sussex.

Publishes a list of UK associations who help allergy sufferers, regu-

194

larly updated and thus particularly useful. 25p brings you a copy of their booklet, *Understanding allergies*.

Foodwatch, High Acre, East Stour, Gillingham, Dorset SP8 5JR. Tel: 0747–85261.

A technical advisory service and supplier of specialized food ingredients. Have a mail-order service and attempt to keep their prices reasonable and stable. They can help customers identify ingredients of other people's manufactured foods.

Foresight (Association for promotion of preconceptual care), The Old Vicarage, Church Lane, Witley, near Godalming, Surrey.

Their *Guidelines for future parents* contains much of interest.

Foundation for the Study of Infant Deaths, 5th Floor, 4 Grosvenor Place, London SW1X 7HD. Tel: 01–235–1731, 01–245–9421

Friends of the Earth Ltd., 9 Poland St, London WIV 3DG. Tel: 01–434–1684, 01–437–6121.

Health Education Council, 78 New Oxford St., London WC1A 1AH. Tel: 01–637–1881.

Hyperactive Children's Support Group (HACSG) for hyperactive, learning disabled, and allergic children. Hon. Chairman: Mrs I.D. Colquhoun, Mayfield House, Yapton Road, Barnham, Bognor Regis, West Sussex, PO22 0BJ.

Journal of Alternative Medicine, 30 Station Approach, West Byfleet, Surrey KT14 6NF.

Medic. Alert Foundation, 9 Hanover St, London WIR 9HF.
for medically accepted identity braclets, etc.

The Migraine Trust 45 Great Ormond St., London WC1N 3HD. Tel: 01–278–2676.

National Association of Parents of Sleepless Children (NAPSC), P.O. Box 38, Prestwood, Great Missenden, Bucks. HP16 O52.

The National Society for Research into Allergy (NSRA), PO Box 45, Hinckley, Leicester LE10 1JY.

Helps allergy sufferers by publishing a Newsletter with useful information, lists, correspondence, news experiences etc. They aim to assist in establishing agreed and well-researched ways of diagnosing and treating allergic illnesses, which can become

Food for thought

accepted parts of every doctor's knowledge. They will help you find medical assistance, too.

National Eczema Society, The General Secretary, Tavistock House North, Tavistock Square, London WC1H 9SR. Tel: 01–388–4097. (SAE, please).

National Society of Non Smokers, 40–48 Hanson St., London WIP 7DE. Tel: 01–636–9103.

National Society for Clean Air, 134, 137 North St., Brighton BN1 1RG. Tel: 0273–26313/4/5.

Non-Smokers' Campaign, 1 Birdbush Ave., Saffron Walden, Essex

Provides a directory of smoke-free restaurants, etc.

Research Group for Autists, 49 Orchard Avenue, Shirley, Croydon CR0 7HE, Surrey.

Encourage neurophysiological and biochemical research into the causes of autism and provide members with latest information.

Schizophrenia Association of Great Britain, Hon. Sec, Mrs. G.P. Hemmings, BSc, Tyr Twr, Llanfair Hall, Caernarvon, Gwynnedd LL5 1TT.

Search for improved treatments for schizophrenia which are curative rather than palliative. Publish Newsletter which examines nutritional as well as drug treatments.

Society for Environmental Therapy, Secretary: Andy Beckingham, 31 Sarah St., Darwen, Lancs, BB3 3ET.

SET investigates the environmental causes of disease, usually focusing on food. Both lay and professional members are encouraged to contribute their ideas to the quarterly Newsletter which features a wide range of reports, scientific articles, suggestions for treatment, and conference reports, etc.

People with chemical sensitivities who need to find less polluted food, should be aware of *The Organic Food Guide* (ed.) A.Gear, published by Henry Doubleday Research Association, Convent Lane, Bocking, Braintree, Essex CM7 6RW.

Steroid Action Aid Group, 35 Lansdown Rd., Seven Kings, Ilford, Essex. Tel: 01–597–0823 office hours, or SAE.

Resources

Self-help group for those taking steroids and suffering side effects.

TALC (Teaching Aids at Low Cost), Institute of Child Health, 30 Guilford St., London WCIN 1EM.

Write for catalogue—excellent materials, unbelievably cheap.

The Vegetarian Society (UK) Ltd., Parkdale, Dunham Road, Altrincham, Cheshire WA14 4QG Tel: 061–928–0793.

53 Marloes Rd., Kensington, London W8 6LA. Tel: 01–937–7739.

I do not recommend vegetarianism for children: any narrowing of the diet may create further nutritional hazards. However, if you wish to be vegetarian—and there are good reasons for that decision too—then you MUST be well informed. Such societies are aware of the hazards and can help you avoid them. Before you do this, however, do read Shinwell's article in *Pediatrics* (1982.) **7014**, 582–6.

Wholefood, 24 Paddington St., London W1. Tel. 01–935–3924.

Has an excellent mail order book service.

Worthing Children's Helpline, 20 Welland Rd., Worthing, W. Sussex

Parent self-help group concerned with allergies and hyperactivity.

(C) Professional addresses

Association of Radical Midwives (ARM) c/o The Secretary, 62 Greetby Hill, Ormskirk, Lancs 139 2DT.

ARM's overall aim is to restore the role of the midwife for the benefit of the childbearing woman and her baby. They publish a quarterly Newsletter. It is also worth knowing that the Royal College of Midwives, 15 Mansfield St., London W1M 0BE publishes an excellent Current Awareness Service, listing recent literature on midwifery. At £5 p.a. subscription, this is an excellent resource.

British Homoeopathic Association, 27a Devonshire Street, London W1N 1RJ. Tel: 01–935–2163.

British Nutrition Foundation, 15 Belgrave Square, London SW1X 8PS. Tel: 01–235–4904.

British Society for Allergy & Clinical Immunology: this year their secretary is C.A. Pickering, MB, MRCP, Withenshaw Hospital,

Food for thought

Manchester 23, and so far as I can discover, enquiries about the BSACI should be referred to him.

The BSACI publish a handbook which contains an up-to-date list of allergy clinics of its members. Your GP should, however, be able to refer patients for testing and/or treatment at these clinics on the NHS, and should know the address of your local clinic.

British Holistic Medicine Society, c/o Dr. Patrick Pietroni, St. Mary's Hospital, London.

British Society for Clinical Ecology, (Sec. Dr. R. Finn), Royal Liverpool Hospital, Prescot Street, Liverpool L7 8XP.

Institute for Complementary Medicine, 21 Portland Place, London W1N 3AF. Tel: 01–636–9543.

Runs the Association for Complementary Medicine, which informs members about complementary medicine and publishes a Newsletter.

National Association of Patient Participation Groups, c/o Hazel Ackerly, 28 Heol-y-Deryn, Glycorrwg, Near Port Talbot, West Glamorgan.

These groups are do-it-together medicine—doctors and patients meeting to develop health services in their local area. SAE.

(D) Breast-feeding support and promotion groups/contacts

Association of Breastfeeding Mothers, 14 Pleasant Grove, Shirley, Croydon, Surrey.

131 Mayow Rd., Sydenham, London SE26 4HZ. Tel: 01–461–0022.

Association for Improvement of Maternity Services, 61 Dartmouth Park Road, London NW 5.

Baby Milk Action Coalition, c/o Patti Rundall, 34 Blinco Grove, Cambridge.

National Childbirth Trust, Breastfeeding Promotion Group, 9 Queensborough Terrace, London W2 3TB. Tel: 01–221–3833

La Leche League (Great Britain), 12 Redvins Halnaker, Chichester, W. Sussex PO18 0QJ.
or
Dept. A. BM 3424, London WCIV 6XX. Tel: 01–404–5011.

Resources

Re-lactation: Ann Buckley, 14 Brookway Grasscroft, Oldham, Lancs. Tel: Saddleworth 2881.

See also *New Generation*, vol. 2, no. 3.

Colgate Medical Ltd., Fairacres Estate, Dedworth Rd., Windsor, Berks, SL4 4LE can ssupply details of their nursing supplementer.

TALC (Teaching Aids at Low Cost), P.O. Box 49, St. Albans, Herts AL1 4AX.

Non-profit group producing books, films, slides, and other teaching aids about health, nutrition, and development. Health workers, CEA, and other groups may find aids useful, even though the primary emphasis is for community health in developing countries. A group worth supporting.

UNICEF (UK Committee), 55 Lincolns Inn Fields, London WC2A 3NB

Some excellent educational materials available write for their catalogue and do read their annual *Report on the State of the Worlds' Children*.

War on Want, 467 Caledonia Road, London N7.

Publishes: *Marketing Infant Formula, an annotated bibliography* (125pp) and others.

Companies supplying breast-feeding resources

Kaneson pumps and plastic bags for human milk:
Kimal Scientific Products Ltd., Unit E, Trading Estate, Uxbridge, Middlesex UR8 2RT.

Pumps, pasteurizering systems, bottles; and nursing supplementers: Colgate Medical Ltd., Fairacres Estate, Dedworth Rd., Windsor, Berks, SL4 4LE (Tel: Windsor 60378). Bottles also available from Natural Joy, 1 Howard Close, London N11 1EH.

Egnell hand pump, and details of electric breast pumps, also available from NCT.

Groups providing postnatal support, whose attitudes to breast-feeding are unknown to me at present:

Association for postnatal illness (postnatal depression), 7 Gowan Ave., Fulham, London SW6. Tel: 01–731–4108.

Food for thought

Crysis (crying babies), c/o Alison Liebeskind, 32 Prince George Ave., London N14 Tel: 01-360-2430.

Meet-a-mum-association, 26A Cumnor Hill, Oxford OX2 9HA (write only; SAE).

Twins Clubs Association, Roma, Grange Rd., Ash, Aldershot, Hants. (write only; SAE).

National Council for the Single Woman and her Dependants, 29 Chilworth Mews, London W2 3RG. Tel: 01-262-1451.

3. OVERSEAS RESOURCES

(A) Allergy and the environment

Australia

Allergy Association, Australia (AAA), PO Box 298, Ringwood, Vic. 3134 Tel: 03-420-5330 office hours.

AAA has many groups around Australia, and is in contact with other interested groups, so it serves as a clearing house for Australian information.

Canada

Allergy Information Association (AIA), Room 7, 25 Poynter Drive, Weston, Ontario M9R 1K8.

An excellent range of inexpensive leaflets. Write for catalogue.

Canadian Schizophrenia Foundation, 2135 Albert St., Regina, Saskatchewan S4P 2V1.

Write for catalogue. Some fascinating material—orthomolecular psychiatry.

Human Ecology Foundation of Canada, 206 St. James St. Sth., Hamilton, Ontario L8P 3A9.

Write for catalogue.

Eire

Asthma Society of Ireland, 24 Anglesea St., Dublin 2. Tel: 716551.

Irish Allergy Association, PO Box 1067, Churchtown, Dublin 14.

Resources

New Zealand

Allergy Awareness Association (Inc.) PO Box 12–701, Penrose, Auckland 6.

Auckland Hyperactivity Association, PO Box 36099, Northcote,Auckland 9.

United States

Allergy Foundation of America, 801Second Ave., New York 10017.

Allergy Foundation of Lancaster Country, Box 1424, Lancaster, Pennsylvania 17604.
Write for catalogue.

Human Ecology Action League (HEAL), 4054 McKinney Ave., Suite 310, Dallas, Texas 75204.
National organization—aims to educate and to secure legislative changes.

L.D. Dickey Enterprises, 635 Gregory Rd., Fort Collins, Colorado 80524.
Good catalogue of clinical ecology books etc. Will mail order.

Society for Clinical Ecology, 1750 Humboldt St., Denver, Colorado 80218.
Provides names of US physicians practising clinical ecology.

For other countries, ask either AAA or AIA for contacts. They have many international members. Please send me new groups or address changes for later editions.

(B) Breast-feeding support and promotion groups around the world

New entries very welcome. If you want to find a group in some place not mentioned, check with either;
Carolyn Tsikouris (LLLI leader responsible for foreign groups), 1039 Brampton Court, Park Forest Sth., IL60466, USA
or
International Breastfeeding Affiliation, P.O. Box 59436, Nairobi, Kenya.

Food for thought

or

Maternal and Child Health Unit, Family Health Division, World Health Organisation, 1211 Geneva 27, Switzerland.
Please let me know if these entries are out of date or incorrect.

Argentina

Nunu Grupo de Ayuda Materna, Av. Maipu 2901 1636 Pcia (Bs. As.) Republica Argentina. Contact: Liliana Carallido.
or
Naipu 1485-I.V. Vicente Lopez, Buenos Aires, Republica Argentina

Australia

NMAA (Nursing Mothers' Association of Australia.) PO Box 231, Nunawading, 3131. Tel: 03–877–5011.
The major breast-feeding organization: 17 000 members and groups all over Australia. Useful pamphlets available.

Parents' Centres Australia (PCA), PO Box 398, Parramatta, 2150. Tel: 02–519–1474.
A group akin to Britain's NCT which is concerned with every aspect of parenting from pregnancy onwards.

IBFAN Australia, c/o Australian Consumers' Association, 57 Carrington Rd., Marrickville, N.S.W. 2204. Tel: 02–558–0099.
Contact Kate Short.

ICEA International Co-ordinator Jan Cornfoot, 42 Lenori Rd., Gooseberry Hill, W.A. 6076
Jan is keen to set up a network of competent people in the field of pregnancy, childbirth, and early parenting, with an awareness of how social practices affect women in Australia and in less-developed countries.

La Leche League Australia, c/o Pinky McKay, 8 Gateshed Drive, Wantirna 3152. Tel: 221–1997.

Bahamas

La Leche League of Bahamas, 1025 Mulberry Court, Fairview, Pa. 16415.
Contact Freida Lukjanczvk.

Resources

Barbados

La Leche League of Barbados, C/-BDD, PO Box 167, Carlisile House, Hincks Street, Bridgetown, Barbados.

Belgium

Borstvoeding Belgie, V.2.W. Borstreiding, Kortehoekstraat 2 d, 9308 Hofstade-Aalst. Tel: 053–78–96–85.

Canada

Infact Canada, 10 Trinity Square, Toronto, Ont. M5G 1B1. Tel: 416–595–9819

Chile

Liga Chilena De La Lactancia Materna, Esmeralda-678-Piso, Santiago-Centro

Costa Rica

Nancy Sabean, APOYO Centre pro-Mujer, Apartado 470, 'San Pedro, Montes de Oca, San Jose, Costa Rica.

Denmark

Ammelauget, Ulla Markussen, Smedevejen 1, DK-4920-Sollosted.

Ammehjaelpen in Denmark, Ellyn Grubbe, Bregningevej 1, Grønnegade, DK-4892 Rettinge. Tel: 03–864533.

Ammeradgivningen i Foraeldre og Fødsel, C/- Anne Olsen, GL Søstvej 142, 6200 Abenrå.

Egypt

Dr El Sayd Abd Allah, Society of Friends of Mothers' Milk, Damietta General Hospital, Maadi Medical Centre, St. 105-Maadi, Cairo.

El Salvador

Calma, Urbanizacion la Esperanza, diagonal, poligono L-Np. 226, San Salvador.

Contact Dr Cristina Villafuerte.

Food for thought

Fiji

Nursing Mothers of Fiji, PO Box 856, Suva.
Contact Christine Weir.

France

Solidarilait, Centre Puercultrice, Ave Brune, Paris 14.

Guatemala

Corsanu, Consultoria Regional de Salud y Nutricion, 8 ave 17–32, zona 1, apto. 225, Guatemala.
Contact Aura M. de Giron, R.. and Ana Aimee de Hacohen.

Honduras

Pro alma, Honduras, PO Box 512, San Pedro. Sula.
Contact Judy Canahuati.

Hong Kong

La Leche League, Hong Kong, c/o Debra Robins, Flat 55, 9th Floor 37 Conduit Rd., Hong Kong

Hong Kong Childbirth Education Group, Sarah Bath, 4 Wavell House, Victoria Barracks, Hong Kong or Jean Luscher, PO Box 819, Hong Kong. Tel: 3–370878.

India

Dr Raj Anand, Consumers' Guidance Society of India, 55 Kair Apts., Worli, Bombay.

Indonesia

Department of Child Health, Udavana University, Denpasar, Bali.
Contact Dr Sudaryat Suraatmaja.

La Leche League of Jakarta, C/- Dumex, PO Box 407, Jakarta.
Contact Jennifer Brinch.

Indonesian Midwives Association, J1. Johar Baru V/13D Kayuawet, Jakarta Pusat.
Contact Mrs Langkay Rambitan.

BK-PP-ASI, B.K.O. Pasi (Working Unit for Promoting the Use of Breast Milk), Jalan Liliroyor, Manado, Sulawesi Jtara.
Contact Dr Indra D. Elita Arif.

Resources

Ireland

Well Woman Centre, 63 Lr. Leeson St., Dublin 2.

Association for Improvement in Maternity Services 48 Wyvern, Killiney Rd., Dublin. Tel: 856947.

The Home Birth Centre, 3 South Terrace, Inchicore, Dublin 8. Tel: 717295.

La Leche League, 12 Rathdown Park, Greystones, co. Wicklow. Tel: 875368.

Italy

Jenny Della Torre, via B. Goldoni 23, Milano 20129.

Japan

Japan CEA, Mitsoo Yamada, 1–16, Yoshikura-cho, Yokosuka City, Kanagawa Pref., Japan 238. Tel: 0468–22–6142.

Kenya

Breastfeeding Information Group, PO Box 59436, Nairobi. Contact Anne Emmesson.

Malaysia

Nursing Mothers Association of Penang, 9 Jalan Chenghai, Tanjong Bungah Tolong, Penang, Malaysia. Contact Rhonda Douglas.

PPPI Malaysian Breastfeeding Advisory Association, 3rd Floor 8, Jalan Klyne, Kuala Lumpur 01–21. Tel: 03–468315; 03–786316.

Consumers' Association of Penang (CAP), 27 Jalan Kelawai, Penang.

International Organisation of Consumer Unions (IOCU) Asia, PO Box 1045, Penang.

Mexico

La Leche League of Mexico City, Mimosas 45, Olivar de los Padres, Mexico 20, D.F. Contact Paulina Smith.

Food for thought

Netherlands

La Leche League of Zoetermeer, Amalia Plaats 30, 2713 B J Zoetermeer.

Contact: Marijke Wisse.

Verenging Borstvoeding Naturlijk (Breastfeeding Naturally), Postbus 119, 3960 BC Wijk bij Duurstede, and Schrikslaan 3,1, 3762 TB Socst a/d Yssel. Tel: 01807–15645; 08376–3317.

Margaret Brethouwer, Korhoenderveld 26, 5431 HH Cuijk.

New Zealand

La Leche League of New Zealand, PO Box 2307, Christchurch.

Contact Rachel Walker.

N.Z. Parents' Centres Federation, 54 Murphy St., Wellington.

Nicaragua

Genesis II, Apartado 2829, Managua

Norway

Ammehjelpen, St Olavs gate 5, Oslo 1, Tel: 02–11–14 70.

Panama

Prolacma Panama, Apartado 6–133, El Dorado, Panama.

Contact Charlotte Elton or Janice Herring.

Panama Canal, PSC Box 2673, APO Miami, FI 34002.

Papua New Guinea

Susu Mamas, Box 5857 Boroko, Papua New Guinea. Tel: Tricia Sangwine, (Port Moresby) 251316.

Peru

Peru-Mujer, Avda. Espana 578 no. 301, Lima 5.

Contact Jeanine Velasco.

Philippines

NMAP-KINA. 66 JP Rizal St., Project 4, Quezon City
or
PO Box EA 471, Ermita, Manila.

Resources

Puerto Rico

Family Centred Education, Calle Rodeno 1565, El Paraiso, Rio Piedras 00926 (Joanne Burris, Tel: 767–5083).

Singapore

Singapore Breastfeeding Mothers' Group, Consumers Association of Singapore, Trade Union House Annexe, Shenton Way, Singapore 0106. Tel: 222–4165.

Solomon Islands

Lukaotem Picanini, c/o Box 390, Honiara.

South Africa

South Africa Breastfeeding Association, 39 Welgelee Rd, Constantia Hills, 7800 Cape Town.
Contact Mrs Sandy Bailey.

Sweden

Gunilla Ivehag, PL 7047 Frammestad, 46500 Nossebro.

Amningshjalpen, Box 20951, S-931 02 Skelleftea. Tel: 0910–19223.

NAFIA, c/o Ingrid Sillén, Asögatan 78, 2 tr, S-11624, Stockholm.

Switzerland

Informationsdienst und Dritte Welt, Postfach 1686, (Monbijoustrasse 31). CH-3000, Berne. Tel: 031–26–12–32/3.

GIFA (Geneva Infant Feeding Association), PO Box 157, 1211 Geneva 19. Tel: 022–989164.

La Leche Liga Schweiz, Postfach 197, Zurich. 8053.

UNICEF, Palais de Nations 1211 Genève 10. See also Witto.

Trinidad and Tobago

Housewives Assocation of Trinidad and Tobago, PO Box 410, Port of Spain, Trinidad and Tobago, W.I.
Contact Mrs H. Brown, Allison White

Food for thought

The Informative Breastfeeding Service, M. Edoel Avenue, Maraval, Trinidad, W.I.

Contact Marilyn Stollmeyer

or

3 Strasser Parkway, Fondes Amandes, St. Anns, Trinidad
Contact Annette Telfer

Karen Milne, 13 Bel View Dr., Bel Air. La Romain, Trinidad, W.I.

United States

ICEA (International Childbirth Education Association), PO Box 20048, Minneapolis MN 55420. Tel: 612–854–8660.

A Federation of groups and individuals interested in family-centred maternity and infant care. Publishes Bookmarks, and runs the ICEA Bookcentre (same address). An excellent source of relevant books. International Co-ordinator

Jan Cornfoot, 42 Lenori Rd., Gooseberry Hill, W.A. 6076, Australia, for non-US enquiries.

La Leche League International Inc., 9616 Minneapolis Ave., Franklin Park, Ilinois 60131.

The senior, biggest and most professional breast-feeding organization in the world. Extensive catalogue for breast-feeing publications, including their own book *The Womanly Art of Breast Feeding* (1981 much improved edition) and cookbook *Whole Foods for the Whole Family,* which uses only unprocessed foods. Some excellent professional materials, including tapes, and *Breastfeeding Abstracts,* a quarterly review of relevant research ($8 annual subscription.)

Health Education Associates Inc., 211 South Easton Rd., Glenside, PA 19038.

Simple, inexpensive leaflets on all aspects of parenting, especially breast-feeding. Write for price list.

Childbirth Graphics. P.O. Box 17025, Irondequoit, Rochester, N.Y. 14617-0325. Excellent materials (some needing revision) on all aspects of birth and feeding. Danner's pamphlets are worth ordering.

Resources

Birth & Life Bookstore, PO Box 70625, Seattle, Washington 98107.

Another first-rate source of cheap US books. Write for catalogue.

Human Lactation Center, 666 Sturges Highway, Connecticut 06880. Tel: 203–259–5995.

While this group, headed by Dr Dana Raphael, publishes some useful and insightful material, its concern for women's rights and 'freedom of choice', and its working relationship with major infant food companies may be the cause of a very odd selection of materials, e.g. in one issue of *The Lactation Review*, the then proposed WHO Code was misrepresented as 'legislating breast-feeding', the Papua New Guinea legislation was criticized as leading to the use of inappropriate feeding bottles without mentioning the dramatic drop in infantile gastroenteritis, etc. Thousands of copies of an earlier issue were widely distributed by formula companies.

Anyone reading *The Lactation Review* or other recent material by Dr Raphael ought to be aware that some of her views are hotly disputed by people such as the Jelliffes, members of the Cornell University Nutrition School, the Population Council, etc. (Unlike her, these people are medically trained—Raphael is an anthropologist, which partly explains her perspective.) It is very necessary to read both sides of this argument before accepting either point of view—situations can be distorted by omitting facts as well as by misrepresenting them. At present Dr Raphael seems to be actively promoting her line through contacts with mother support groups, some of whom may be unaware of the controversies (cf. *Congressional Record,* July 25, 1979, p. E3866–70). It seems to me highly likely that the uncritical acceptance of Dr Raphael's arguments will lead to less breast-feeding rather than more, whatever her avowed aim.

Lact-Aid International, P.O. Box 1066, Athens, TN 37303. Tel: 615–7449090.

A few good monographs, many taken from *Keeping Abreast Journal*, and information about Lact-Aid, which the Averys developed.

Center for Science in the Public Interest, 1779 Church St. N.W., Washington DC 20036.

Nutritional Sciences, Cornell University, Savage Hall, Ithaca, NY 14853.

Food for thought

Publishes the results of research into breast-feeding around the world—cf. Bibliography.

Formula, PO Box 39051, Washington DC 20016.

Group concerned with the impact of chloride-deficient formulae. Send stamped envelope and $2 (US) for information.

IBFAN (International Babyfoods Action Network), 310 E. 38th St., Suite 310, Minneapolis, MN 55409.

Much material, including *Breast is Best-from Policy to Practice Action Pack.* (Also available from GIFA and War on Want.)

Interfaith Centre on Corporate Responsibility (ICCR), 475 Riverside Drive, Rm 566, New York NY 10027.

International Nutrition Communication Service, Education Development Center, 55 Chapel St., Newton, MA 02160. Tel: 617–969–7100.

The Population Council, One Dag Hammarskjold Plaza, New York, NY 10017.

Publishes *Studies in Family Planning,* free issue on breast-feeding.

Population Information Program, Johns Hopkins University, 426 North Broadway, Baltimore, MD 21205.

Reports on many aspects of fertility, including breast-feeding, and health (ORT, tobacco, etc.).

UNICEF, 866 UN Plaza, New York, NY 10017.

Excellent educational materials including slides, tapes for radio spots, etc.

Vanuatu (Previously New Hebrides)

Mrs. C. Kirkpatrick, PO Box 257, Port Vila, New Hebrides, South Pacific.

Venezuela

Edificio Oriente, Avenida 5 de Julio, Puerto la Cruz.

West Germany

Arbeitsgemeinschaft Freier Stillgruppen, C/- Sylvia Brunn, Am Bruckenberg 6, 5307 Wachtberg Oberbachem. Tel: 0228–34–22–48.

Resources

Zimbabwe

La Leche League Umtali, 46 Kingfisher Street, Greenside, Umtali.
Contact Mrs. Desma Noland Evans

La Leche League of Marlborough, 3 Mansfield Rd., Marlborough, Salisbury.
Contact Nikki Galbraith.

La Leche League Highlands, 9 Parkham Road, PO Chisipite, Salisbury.
Contact Joanne Fletcher.

La Leche League Avondale-Emerald Hill, 'The End' Serendip Close, Emerald Hill, Salisbury.

Envoi

As victims of environmentally induced disease, you have embarked on a process of self-education which could change many of your perspectives on health and food. You may come to see the extent of the problems that have been created over many years in our affluent society by a combination of ignorance, carelessness, commercial pressures, public apathy, and blind faith in 'scientific' progress. You are about to learn how difficult it can be to find relatively uncontaminated, reliably labelled, basic foods. (The cost will be beyond some of you, unless a food co-operative is to be found nearby.) You may begin to discover more and more that is frightening in the manufacture, use, and disposal of many products that you once took for granted. Your new awareness of how our total environment affects us will impose a burden of responsibility that we would all rather live without. But our children's children may not be able to live at all if we choose to ignore that burden, and take no positive action to change even a little of the problems that confront us.

And in this world of global pollution and exported hazards, we can't afford simply to cultivate our own garden. Consider how much worse these problems are in cultures and countries whose basic economy is distorted by the pressures of international consumerism and whose people lack the leverage of money, time, and education. We are responsible for the decline of breast-feeding in the Third World, however indirectly; we are responsible for much more as well. (Subscribe to *New Internationalist*, or send for Friends of the Earth's *Food Politics Primer* and you'll see what I mean.) The decline of breast-feeding has meant the increased incidence of disease everywhere; for Third World countries it means increased foreign debts and increased birth rates as well as increased infant mortality on a monstrous scale. Where thousands of British children may die needlessly, or be learning-disabled, Third World children die by the millions and are irreparably brain-damaged—their mothers endure more pregnancies and die younger too.

My hope is that some of you who benefit by what has been written in this booklet will find that more of your resources of time, energy, and money are being spent on making this one small planet a safer place for all the world's children. I have been enormously encouraged by becoming involved in this work: there is a vast army of caring people in this field of maternal and child health, and a very supportive international network has been created. As the executive director of UNICEF points out, we can bring about change, and soon—or, by ignoring the issue, we can remain part of the problem, not become part of the solution. What you and I do may not be a spectacular—write a letter here, monitor the WHO Code locally, help another mother breast-feed, donate to aid agencies, buy UNICEF cards, reduce our consumption of the world's resources—but we must be convinced that in the developed world, what we do, how we live, DOES matter.

Bibliography

Interested parents who want to learn more, or who want to set up a co-operative library, should read this carefully. The titles listed cover the whole range of family concerns, since problems of food tolerance cannot be dealt with in isolation. Because this is a book written for a wide audience, I have not listed everything I have read, but merely a selection of the items used in originally writing it, together with more recent interesting work. My choice is naturally biased towards those articles or books that most accurately reflect parental experience, which for me remains the touchstone against which academic research is judged. However, there are plenty of opposing views represented in this list as well, and I think it fair to say that anyone who had read most of this literature would have a fairly sound grasp both of what is acceptable and what is controversial in this field. Some of the books are listed because they contain useful bibliographies in their special areas. Naturally, I do not agree with much that they contain.

Before buying, remember that local libraries will get in books, and that good specialist bookstores will almost always send you books on approval.

Allen, D.H. *et al.* (1983). Monosodium-glutamate-induced asthma. (Abstract) *J. Allergy Clin. Immunology.* **71**, 98.

Allergy Information Association (Canada) (1983). *The allergy cookbook.* Methuen, Toronto.

Almroth, S. and Latham, M.C. (1983). Breastfeeding practices in rural Jamaica. *J. Trop. Pediatr.* **28**, 103–9.

Alun-Jones, V. McLaughlan, P., *et al.* (1983) Food intolerance: a major factor in the pathogenesis of irritable bowel syndrome. *Lancet* **ii**, 1115–18.

American Academy of Allergy and Immunology Committee on Adverse Reactions to Foods/National Institute of Allergy and Infectious Diseases (1984). *Adverse reactions to foods.* US Dept. of Health and Human Services, NIH publication no. 84–2442.

Anderson, T.A. (1977). Commercial infant foods: content and composition. *Pediatr. Clin. N. Am.* **24**, 37–47.

Anderson, S. Chinn, H. and Fisher, K. (1982). History and current status of infant formulas. *Am. J. Clin. Nutr.* **35**, 381–97.

Apple, R.D. (1980). 'To be used only under the direction of a physician': commercial infant feeding and medical practice, 1870–1940. *Bull. Hist. Med.* **54**, 402–17.

Arnon, S. (1984). Breastfeeding and toxigenic bacterial infections: missing links in crib death? *Rev. Infect. Dis.* **6**, suppl. 1, 193–201.

Ashby, H.T. (1929). Acute sensitisation in an infant to cows' milk protein. *Arch. Dis. Childn.* IV, 264–9. [This and reports like Cumming (1928) and Tallerman (1934) in the literature seem never to have been noticed.]

Food for thought

Asnes, R.S. and Mones, R.L. (1983). Infantile colic: a review. *J. Dev. Behavioural Pediatr.* **4**, 57–62.

Assignment Children special issue, Breastfeeding and infant health. (1981). [Available through UNICEF or direct from Assignment Children, Villa Le Bocage, Palais des Nations, Geneve 10, Switzerland.]

Atherton, D.J. (1983). The role of foods in atopic eczema. *Clin. Exp. Dermatol.* **8**, 227–32.

Auricchio, S. *et al.* (1983). Does breastfeeding protect against the development of clinical symptoms of coeliac disease in children? *J. Pediatr. Gastroent. Nutr.* **2**, 8–33.

Avery, J.L. (1978). *Induced lactation.* [Available through breastfeeding support groups.]

Aynsley-Green, A. (1983). Hormones and postnatal adaptation to enteral nutrition. *J. Pediatr. Gastroent. Nutr.* **2**, 418–28.

Bahna, S. and Heiner, D.C. (1980). *Allergies to milk.* Grune and Stratton, New York [An excellent review, whose perspectives are being further validated by more recent publications.]

Bahna, S.L. and Gandhi, M.D. (1983). Milk hypersensitivity. 1. Pathogenesis and symptomatology.; 2. Practical aspects of diagnosis, treatment and prevention. *Ann. Allergy.* **50**, 218–23; **50**, 293–301.

Bahna, S.L. and Furakawa, C.T. (1983). Food allergy: diagnosis and treatment. *Ann. Allergy.* **51**, 574–80.

Baldo, B. and Wrigley, C. (1984). Allergy in Australia: symptom, diagnosis and treatment. *Med. J. Aust. 1* **41**, special supplement.

Barnes, P.J. (1984). Nocturnal asthma: mechanisms and treatment. *Br. med. J.* **288**, 1397–8.

Barnetson, R.S. (1981). Late onset atopic eczema and multiple food allergies after infective mononucleosis. *Br. med. J.* **283**, 1086–7.

Baylis, J.M., *et al* (1983). Persistent nausea and food aversions in pregnancy: a possible association with cows' milk allergy in infants. *Clin. Allergy.* **13**, 263–9.

Bentley, D., *et al.* (1984). Abdominal migraine and food sensitivity in children. *Clin. Allergy.* **14**, 499–500.

Bentley, S.J., Pearson, D.J. and Rix, K. (1983). Food hypersensitivity in irritable bowel syndrome. *Lancet* **ii**, 294–7.

Berg, N.O., Jakobsson, I. and Lindberg, T. (1979). Do pre- and post-challenge intestinal biopsies help to diagnose cows' milk protein intolerance? *Acta Paediatr. Scand.* **68**, 657–61.

Berman, B.A. and MacDonnell, K.F. (1981). *Differential diagnosis and treatment of pediatric allergy.* Little, Brown and Co., Boston.

Bienenstock, J. (1984). Mucosal barrier functions. *Nutr. Rev.* **42**, 105–9. [This issue has several other articles of interest.]

Birth and the Family Journal (1981). 8, Special issue, Breastfeeding in post-industrial society.

Bock, S.A. and Martin, M. (1983). The incidence of adverse reactions to foods. (Abstract) *J. Allergy Clin. Immunol.* **71**, 37.

—— (1982). The natural history of food sensitivity. *J. Allergy Clin. Immunol.* **69**, 173–7.

214

Bibliography

Brenemann, J.C. (1983). Overview of food allergy: Historical perspectives. *Ann. Allergy* **51**, 2 pt. 2, 220–1.

Brostoff, J. and Challacombe, S.J. (1982). Food Allergy. *Clinics in immunology and allergy*. W.B. Saunders, Philadelphia.

Buisseret, P.D. (1982). Allergy. *Scientific American* **246**, 82–91.

Buist, R. (1984). *Food intolerance: what it is and how to cope with it* Harper and Row, Sydney [Some good points, but weakest on infant feeding and recommends rotation diets. Useful recipes.]

Bullen, C.L. and Willis, A.T. (1971). Resistance of the breastfed infant to gastroenteritis. *Br. Med. J.* **273**, 338–43.

Burr, M.L. (1983). Does infant feeding affect the risk of allergy? *Arch. Dis. Childn.* **58**, 561–5.

—— (1983). Food intolerance: a community survey. *Br. J. Nutr.* **49**, 417.

Businco, L., *et al.* (1982). Results of a milk and/or egg free diet in children with atopic dermatitis. *Allergol. Immunopathol.* (Madr.) **10**, 283–6.

—— (1983). Prevention of atopic disease in 'at risk' newborns by prolonged breastfeeding *Ann. Allergy* **51**, 296–9.

Butler, J.E. (1979). Immunologic aspects of breast feeding, anti-infectious activity of breast milk. *Semin. Perinatol.* **3**, 255–70.

Caffrey, E.A., *et al.* (1981). Thrombocytopenia caused by cows' milk. *Lancet* (letter) **ii**, 316.

Campbell, N. (1981). Nutritional and immunological benefits of breastfeeding. *Aust. Nurses' J.* **10**, 40–7.

Cant. A.J. *et al.* (1984). Food hypersensitivity made life-threatening by ingestion of asprin. *Br. Med. J.* **288**, 6419, 755–6. [See also articles with Heppell (1984) and Kilshaw (1985).]

Challacombe, D.N. and Baylis, J.M. (1980). Childhood coeliac disease is disappearing (letter) *Lancet* **ii**, 1360.

Chalmers, I. (1983). Scientific enquiry and authoritarianism in perinatal care and education. *Birth* **10**, 151–64. [Required reading!]

Chandra, R.K. (1983). Nutrition immunity and infection: present knowledge and future directions. *Lancet* **i**, 688–91.

—— (ed.) (1984). *Food intolerance.* Elsevier Science Publishing, Amsterdam. [A very useful medical text whose major defect is the almost complete absence of discussion of prophylactic measures and infant feeding.]

Charles, G.A. (1985). Do detergent residues damage the gut? (letter) *Lancet* **i**, 165.

Chin, K.C., *et al.* (1983). Allergy to cows milk presenting as chronic constipation. *Br. med. J.* **287**, 1593.

Chunn, J. (1982). Diagnostic tests for allergy: principles and pitfalls. *Patient Management.* March, pp. 65–73.

Coca, A.F. (1979). *The pulse test.* Arco Publishing Inc., New York.

Coello-Ramirez, P. and Larossa-Harp, A. (1983). Gastrointestinal occult hemorrhage and gastroduodenitis in cows' milk protein intolerance. *J. Pediatr. Gastroent. nutr.* **2**, 215.

Conrad, M.C. (1975). *Allergy cooking.* Pyramid Books, New York.

Cook, P.S. (1978). Child-rearing and mental health. *Med. J. Aust.* **65**, 2, Special supplement, 12 Aug.

Food for thought

Coombs, R.R.A. (1982). The enigma of cot death: is the modified anaphylaxis hypothesis an explanation in some cases? *Lancet* **i**, 1388–9.

Correa, P., *et al.* (1983). Passive smoking and lung cancer. *Lancet* **ii**, 595–7.

Crayton, J.W. (1981). Epilepsy precipitated by food sensitivity: report of a case with double-blind placebo-controlled assessment. *Clin. Electroencephalogr.* **12**, 192–8.

Crook, W. (1975). Food Allergy, the great masquerader. *Ped. Clin. N. Am.* **22**, 229–38.

—— (1980). *Tracking down hidden food allergy.* Professional Books, Jackson, Tennessee. [Cartoon, large-print format. Necessarily over-simplified and could be up-dated, but excellent for those who would find this book heavy going.]

—— (1983). *The yeast connexion.* Professional Books, Jackson, TN. [An exhaustive review of the thrush/candida problem. Controversial, but has certainly helped some people.]

Cruz, J.R., *et al.* (1981). Food antibodies in milk from Guatemalan women. *J. Pediatr.* **99**, 600–2.

Cumming, W.M. (1928). Extreme hypersensitiveness to cows' milk protein in an infant. *Arch. Dis. Child.* **III**, 296–9.

Cunningham. A.S. (1981). Breastfeeding and morbidity in industrialised countries: an up-date. in Jelliffe and Jelliffe, (1981).

—— (1984). Letter. *World Health Forum* **5**, 39.

Curtis-Jenkins, G.H. (1981). Letter. *Lancet* **ii**, 418–19.

Dannaeus, A. and Johansson, S. (1979). A follow-up study of infants with adverse reactions to cows' milk. *Acta Paediatr. Scand.* **689**, 337–82.

—— (1983). Management of food allergy in infancy. *Ann. Allergy* **51**, 303–6. [This issue contains many articles of interest.]

—— (1984). Diet in asthma in infancy and childhood. *Eur. J. Respir. Dis.* **136**, Suppl., 165–7. [This issue has many other articles of interest.]

David, T.J. *et al.* (1984). Nutritional hazards of elimination diets in children with atopic eczema. *Arch. Dis. Child.* **59**, 323–5. Letters, (1984) **59**, 1197; (1985) **60**, 183–4.

Davidson, G.P. *et al.* (1984). Bacterial contamination of the small intestine as an important cause of chronic diarrhoea and abdominal pain: diagnosis by breath hydrogen test. *Pediatrics* **74**, 229–35.

Day, R.L. (1981). Faith, doubt and statistics. *Pediatrics* **67**, 101–6.

Delire, M. *et al.* (1978). Circulating immune complexes in infants fed on cows' milk. *Nature, Lond.* **273**, 632.

Denman, A.M. (1983). Food allergy. *Br. med. J.* **286**, 1164–6.

——, Mitchell, B. and Ansell, B.M. (1983). Joint complaints and food allergic disorders. *Ann. Allergy* **51**, 260–3.

Denning, D.W. and Vijeratnam, R. (1985). Colouring agents in medicine for asthmatic children. (Letter.) *Lancet* **i**, 461–2.

Du Mont, G.C. *et al.* (1984). Gastrointestinal permeability in food-allergic eczematous children. *Clin. Allergy* **14**, 55–9.

Dugdale, A.E. (1981). Infant feeding and child health. *Med. J. Aust.* **2**, 107.

Bibliography

—— (1982). Science and W.H.O. breast milk policy. (Letter.) *Lancet* **ii**, 1105. [Reply by Porter, (**ii**, 1404) stressed the obvious but overlooked fact that the onus of proving safety ought to be on those who propose radical departures from physiological norms, not those who advocate normal feeding. See also discussion in *World Health Forum*, (1984) **5**, 37–9, 145–7.]

Eagle, R. (1979). *Eating and allergy.* Futura Books, London [Easy to read overview. Useful appendices on hidden foods, food families, good historical perspective.]

Eastham, E.J. and Walker, W.A. (1980). Adverse effects of milk ingestion on the gastrointestinal tract—an update. *Gastroenterology* **76**, 365–74.

Eaton, K. (1982). *Pocket guide to allergies.* Arlington Books, London. [A useful mini-guide.]

Ebrahim, G.J. (1980). *Breastfeeding, the biological option.* Macmillan, London.

—— (1978). *A handbook of tropical paediatrics.* Macmillan, London.

—— (1983). *Nutrition in mother and child health.* Macmillan, London. [Excellent basic books, with a suitably sceptical approach to the question of artificial feeding. Good treatment of diagnosis of growth retardation. Although designed for situations in developing countries, these are very useful primary health resources anywhere.]

Edmeades, R. *et al.* (1981). Infantile gastroenteritis—relationship between cause, clinical course and outcome. *Med. J. Aust.* **2**, 29–32.

Egger, J. *et al.* (1983). Is migraine food allergy? *Lancet* **ii**, 865–8.

—— (1985). Controlled trial of oligoantienic diet in the hyperkinetic syndrome. *Lancet* **i**, 540–5. [These studies are essential reading. They confirm the individuality of response in time, dose, symptoms, duration; the existence of withdrawal symptoms; the benefits of dietary exclusion in inducing greater tolerance; the interaction with non-dietary excitants; the difficulty of standardized challenge regimes; and the benefit to patients with symptoms as varied as migraine, epilepsy, and hyperkinesis. Studies which do not take such trouble are likely not to produce such spectacular results.]

Ellis, E.F. (ed.) (1983). Symposium on pediatric allergy. *Ped. Clin. N. Am.* **30**, 5.

Evans, J. (1979). Effects of chemicals. [Talk given 28 May; available from CASA, (Congenital Abnormality Support Association), 7 Loongana Avenue, Oak Park, Victoria 3046, Australia.]

Falkner, F. and Kretchmer, N. (1985). (ed.) Workshop on introduction of food to infants. *Am. J. Clin. Nutr.* **41**, 381–510. [Another interesting collection of papers of varying quality, with some disturbing features. To be read with critical faculties well honed.]

Fallstrom, S.P. *et al.* (1984). Influence of breast feeding on the development of cows' milk protein antibodies and the IgE level. *Int. Archs. appl. Immun.* **75**, 87–91. [Confirming benefits of breastfeeding and prolonged weaning.]

Food for thought

Farah, D.A. *et al.* (1985). Specific food intolerance: its place as a cause of gastrointestinal symptoms. *Gut* **26**, 164–8.

Feigal, R.J. (1981). Dental caries potential of liquid medication. *Pediatrics* **68**, 418–19.

Ferguson, A. (1985). Immunological response to food. *Proc. Nutr. Soc.* **44**, 73–80. [Part of a symposium on Nutritional Aspects of Normal and Pathological Gut Function, reproduced in full in this issue.]

Fergusson, D.M. *et al.* (1983). Asthma and infant diet. *Arch. Dis. Child.* **58**, 48–51. [Faulty study design, surely! Apart from retrospectivity, the groups compared were either breast milk alone to 4 months, or any other combination of breast and bottle feeding. So the child exclusively breast-fed until 15 weeks is averaged with the totally bottle-fed. Kajosaari (1983) also makes it clear that 4 months is too early for maximum prophylactic benefits of breast-feeding. And unless studies are prospective there is no hope of controlling the odd bottle or tiny taste given by well-meaning others.]

Firer, M.A. *et al.* (1981). Effect of antigen load on the development of milk antibodies in infants allergic to milk. *Br. med. J.* **283**, 693–6.

Fisher, C. (1981). Breast-feeding: a midwife's view. *J. Mat. Child Health.* February, pp. 52–7.

Fishaut, M. *et al.* (1981). Bronchomammary axis in the response to RSV. *J. Pediatr.* **99**, 186–91.

Fisons Limited. (1980). *Proceedings of the first food allergy workshop.* Medical Education Services, Oxford.

—— (1983). *Proceedings of the second Fisons food allergy workshop.* Medical Education Services, Oxford. [These can be obtained from Fisons, together with a publication called *It's something you ate*, which gives details about diets. Write to Pharmaceutical Division, Derby Rd., Leicestershire, LE11 0BB.]

Fomon, S.J. *et al.* (1981). Cows' milk feeding in infancy—GI blood loss and iron nutritional status. *J. Pediatr.* **98**, 540–5.

Ford, R.P. *et al.* (1983). Cows' milk hypersensitivity: immediate and delayed onset clinical patterns. *Arch. Dis. Child.* **58**, 856–62. [This covers much of the talk given at the seminar on cows' milk intolerance, November 1982, referred to in the text.]

Foresight (1981) *Guidelines for future parents* (see p. 195).

Forman, R. (1980). *How to control your allergies.* Larchmont Books, New York.

Frank, A.L. *et al.* (1982). Breastfeeding and respiratory virus infection. *Pediatrics* **70**, 239. (Correspondence, **71**, 470.)

Frazier, C.A. (1980). *Coping and living with allergies.* Prentice Hall, Englewood Cliffs, New Jersey. [First rate; good illustrations and summaries.]

Freed, D.L.J. (ed.) (1984). *The health hazards of milk.* Baillière Tindall, London. [Interesting papers, with formula apologists pushing a line as strongly as clinicians and researchers who question the value of milk in Western diet.]

Freier, S. and Eidelman, A. (ed.) (1980). *Human milk, its biological and*

Bibliography

social value. Excerpta Medica, Amsterdam.

Garza, C. (1984). The unique values of human milk. in *Report* of the Surgeon General's Workshop on Breastfeeding and Human Lactation. [See Koop (1984) Gaul, G.E. (1982) Human milk as food. in Milunsky *et al.*]

—— (1985). Significance of growth modulators in human milk. In Proceedings Workshop on Current Issues in Feeding the Normal Infant. *Pediatrics* **75**, suppl., 135–214. [Some excellent papers, but there are some puzzling aspects about this (as also some other recent meetings) that I shall be looking into.]

Gerrard, J.W. (ed.) (1980). *Food allergy.* C.C. Thomas, Springfield, Illinois. [Essential reading, particularly if interested in renal, cardiovascular, and CNS effects of foods, which have not been emphasized elsewhere.]

—— (1983). Sensitisation to substances in breast milk: recognition, management and significance. *Ann. Allergy* **51**, 2 pt. 2, 300–2.

—— (1984). Allergies in breastfed babies to foods ingested by the mother. *Clin. Rev. Allergy* **2**, 143–9. [An excellent summary article, in an issue which is required reading.]

Gibson, R.A. and Kneebone, G.M. (1981). Fatty acid composition of infant formulae. *Austr. Paediatr. J.* **17**, 46–53.

Gillin, F.D. *et al.* (1983). Human milk kills parasitic intestinal protozoa. *Science* **221**, 1290–2.

Glaser, J. (1955). The prophylaxis of allergic disease with special reference to the newborn infant. *New York State Med. J.* Sept. 15, pp. 2599–2605.

—— (1975). Intra-uterine sensitisation and allergy in the new-born breastfed infant. *Ann. Allergy* **35**, 256–7.

Glomset, J.A. (1985). Fish, fatty acids and human health. *N. Engl. J. Med.* **312**, 1253–4.

Glynn, M. (1985). Food allergy—fact or fancy? *J. Roy. Soc. Med.* **78**, 265–7.

Golos, N. and Golbitz, F. (1978). *Coping with your allergies.* Simon and Schuster, New York. [Excellent for environmental changes.]

Gordon, R.R. *et al.* (1982). IgE and eczema-asthma syndrome in early childhood. *Lancet*, **i**, 72–5. [Criticized, *Lancet* **i**, 339 (1982).]

Graham, J. (1981). *Multiple sclerosis.* Thorsons Publishers, Wellingborough, Northamptonshire.

Grant, J. (1984). *The state of the world's children.* Oxford University Press. [These UNICEF annual reports should be required reading for everyone.]

Greiner, T. (1979). Methodological pitfalls in breastfeeding studies. *J. trop. Pediatr. Environ. Child Health.* Feb., pp. 1–2.

Gruskay, F.L. (1982). Comparison of breast, cow, and soy milk feedings in the prevention of the onset of allergic diseases: a 15 year prospective study. *Clin. Pediatr.* **21**, 486–91.

Gryboski, J. and Walker, W.A. (1983). *Gastrointestinal problems in the infant.* W.B. Saunders, Philadelphia.

219

Food for thought

Gurwitz, D. *et al.* (1981). Increased incidence of bronchial reactivity in children with a history of bronchiolitis in infancy. *J. Pediatr.* **98**, 551.

Hagelburg, S. *et al.* (1982). The protein tolerance of VLBW infants fed human milk protein-enriched mother's milk. *Acta Paediatr. Scand.* **71**, 597–601.

Hambraeus, L. (1977). Proprietary milk versus human milk in infant feeding. *Pediatr. Clin. N. Am.* **24**, 17–36.

Hamburger, R.N. *et al.* (1983). Current status of the clinical and immunologic consequences of a prototype allergic disease prevention program. *Ann. Allergy* **51**, 281–90.

Hardyment, C. (1983). *Dream babies: child care from Locke to Spock.* Jonathon Cape, London; Oxford University Press paperback. [A wonderful book—the perfect present for new parents. Entertaining, informative, and liberating.]

Harrison, M. *et al.* (1976). Cows' milk protein intolerance: a possible association with gastroenteritis, lactose intolerance, and IgA deficiency. *Br. Med. J.* **1**, 1501–4.

Hathaway, M.J. and Warner, J.O. (1983). Compliance problems in the dietary management of eczema. *Arch. Dis. Child.* **58**, 463–4. [Compliance rates were much better in the Egger studies; there is certainly need for follow-up support and practical help.]

Hattevig, G. *et al* (1984). Clinical symptoms and IgE responses to common food proteins in atopic and healthy children. *Clin. Allergy* **14**, 551–9.

Heiner, D.C. (1984). Modern research relating to food allergy and its implications, *Clin. Rev. Allergy* **2**, 1–5. [Essential reading.]

Helsing, E. (1984). Feeding practices in Europe: beliefs and motivations— and possibilities for change. *J. Trop. Pediatr.* **30**, 244–51.

Hemmings, W.A. (1981). Letter. *Lancet* **ii**, 261.

Heppell, L.M.J. *et al.* (1984). Reduction in the antigenicity of whey proteins by heat treatment: a possible strategy for producing a hypoallergenic infant milk formula. *Br. J. Nutr.* **51**, 29–36.

Herbst, J. (1981). Gastro-oesophageal reflux. *J. Pediatr.* **98**, 859.

Hide, D.W. and Guyer, B.M. (1981). Clinical manifestations of allergy related to breast and cows' milk feeding. *Arch. Dis. Child.* **56**, 172–5.

—— (1982). Prevalence of infant colic. *Arch. Dis. Child.* **57**, 559–60.

Hill, D.J. *et al.* (1984). A study of 100 infants and young children with cows' milk allergy. *Clin. Rev. Allergy* **2**, 143–9.

Hills, H.C. (1980). *Good food, milk-free, grain-free.* Keats publishing Company, New Canaan, Connecticutt.

Horgan, B. (1982). *Arthritis in children.* Fontana/Collins, Melbourne. [Unaware of the relevance of food intolerance research, but otherwise a splendid book.]

Huang, A.S. and Fraser, W.M. (1984). Are sulfite additives really safe? *N. Engl J. Med.* **311**, 542.

Hughes, E.C. *et al.* (1982). Food sensitivity in attention-deficit-disorder with hyperactivity. *Ann. Allergy* **49**, 276–80.

Hunter, J. (1985). Irritable bowel syndrome. *Proc. Nutr. Soc.* **44**, 141–3.

Bibliography

[Compliance rates were excellent, as was long-term benefit. Other articles of interest in this issue.]

Ibero, M. *et al.* (1982). Dyes, preservatives and salicylates in the induction of food intolerance and/or hypersensitivity in children. *Allergol. Immunopathol.* (Madr.) **10**, 263–8.

International Confederation of Midwives (1984). *Breastfeeding: a challenge for midwives.* [Report of a workshop. Available from ICM., 57 Lower Belgrave St., London, SW1W0LR.]

Isbister, C. (1979). *Should I call the doctor?* Sphere Books, Melbourne.

Iyngkaran, N. *et al.* (1979). Cows' milk protein sensitive enteropathy—an important cause of protracted diarrhoea in infancy. *Austr. Paediatr. J.* **15**, 266–70.

Jackson, P.G. *et al.* (1981). Intestinal permeability in patients with eczema and food allergy. *Lancet* **i**, 1285–6.

Jackson, R.T. *et al.* (1982). Mortality from asthma: a new epidemic in New Zealand. *Br. med. J.* **285**, 771–4.

Jackson, W. Gracey, M. and Anderson, C. (1983). How should we manage acute diarrhoea? *Medicine Forum.* Sydney. [Available, with additional material, from USV Pharmaceuticals, 172 Princes Highway, Arncliffe, NSW 2205.]

Jakobsson, I. and Lindberg, T. (1978). Cows' milk as a cause of colic in breastfed infants. *Lancet* **ii**, 437.

—— (1979). A prospective study of cows' milk protein intolerance in Swedish infants. *Acta Paediatr. Scand.* **68**, 853–9.

—— (1983). Cows' milk proteins cause colic in breastfed infants: a double-blind cross-over study. *Pediatrics* **71**, 268–9. [See also Evans (1981) and Lothe (1982) and *Lancet* letters, (1981) **ii**, 261; *Lancet* (1981) **ii**, 418–19.]

Jarrett, E. and Hall E. (1979). Selective suppression of IgE antibody responsiveness by maternal influence. *Nature, Lond.* **280**, 145–6.

Jelliffe, D.B. and Jelliffe, E.F.P. (ed.) (1978). *Human milk in the modern world.* Oxford University Press. [Absolutely essential text for anyone concerned with any aspect of infant feeding. Cheap ELBS version available for developing countries.]

—— (1982). *Adverse effects of foods.* Plenum Press, New York [Excellent text for putting intolerance problems into context.]

—— (1981–3). *Advances in international maternal and child health*, Vols. 1–3. Oxford University Press. [This is an important series, although its expense renders it out of range for many who would otherwise read it. More fully reviewed in my next book.]

—— (1982). *Nutrition and growth.* Plenum Press, New York.

Jemmott, J.B. *et al.* (1983). Academic stress, power motivation, and decrease in secretion rate of salivary secretory IgA. *Lancet* **i**, 1400–2.

Jenkins, H.R. *et al.* (1984). Food allergy: the major cause of infantile colitis. *Arch Dis. Child.* **59**, 326–9.

Johnstone, D.C. *et al.* (1975). Factors associated with the development of asthma and hay-fever in children: the possible risks of hospitalisation, surgery, and anesthesia. *Pediatrics* **56**, 579–85.

Food for thought

Johnstone, D.E. (1978). Diagnostic methods in food allergy in children. *Ann. Allergy.* **40**, 110–3.

—— (1981). Current concepts in the natural history of allergic disease in children. *Ann. Allergy* **47**, 225–32.

Jolly, H. (1979). *Book of child care.* Sphere Books, Melbourne.

Jones, S. (1983). *Crying baby, sleepless nights.* Warner Books, New York. [The 1985 edition produced by Thomas Nelson Australia has been fully up-dated, and is preferable to the US edition; but this is an excellent book in any edition.]

Kajosaari, M. and Saarinen, U. (1983). Prophylaxis of atopic disease by six months' total solid food elimination. Evaluation of 135 exclusively breastfed infants of atopic families. *Acta Paediatr. Scand.* **72**, 411–14.

—— (1982). Food allergy in Finnish children aged 1 to 6 years. *Acta Paediatr. Scand.* **71**, 815–19.

Kalveram, K.J. and Forck, G. (1984). Development of pollinosis after ingestion of pollen. *Allergol. Immunopathol.* (Madr.) **22**, 189–92.

Katz, A.J. *et al.* (1984). Milk-sensitive and eosinophilic gastroenteropathy: similar clinical features with contrasting mechanisms and clinical course. *J. Allergy Clin. Immunology* **74**, 72–8.

Keller, M. *et al.* (1985). IgD in human colostrum. *Ped. Res.* **19**, 122–6.

Kemp, A. (1984). The role of allergens in atopic disease in childhood. *Austr. Paediatr. J.* **20**, 161–8. [A useful review of the 'acceptable' position in Australia; omits Kajosaari and Saarinen's post-1980 work and can be criticized in other areas.]

Khin-Maung-U *et al.* (1985). Effect on clinical outcome of breastfeeding during acute diarrhoea. *Br. med. J.* **290**, 587–9. [Babies do better, naturally!]

Kidd, J.M. *et al.* (1983). Food-dependent exercise-induced anaphylaxis. *J. Allergy Clin. Immunol.* **71**, 407–11.

Kilmartin, A. (1980). *Cystitis, a complete self-help guide.* Hamlyn, London. [Another basic book for every parent. Knowing what it contains will prevent many serious problems from ever starting.]

Kilshaw, P.J. and Cant, A.J. (1985). The passage of maternal dietary proteins into human breast milk. *Int. Archs. appl. Immun.* **75**, 8–15.

Kirkland, J. (1985). *Crying and babies: helping families cope.* Croom Helm, London. [A must for all professionals who counsel parents; many parents will also find it helpful, though it is less chatty than Jones (1983). Don't bother with any other books about infant crying—these are the best to date.]

Kjellman, N. (1979). Soy versus cows' milk in infants with a bi-parental history of atopic disease: development of atopic disease and immunoglobulins from birth to 4 years of age. *Clin. Allergy* **9**, 347–58.

Klagsburn, M. *et al.* (1979). Mitogenic activity of human breast milk. *J. Surg. Res.* **26**, 417–22.

Klein, V.L. *et al.* (1984). Fetal distress during a maternal systemic allergic reaction. *Obstet. Gynecol.* **64**, (3 Suppl.) 15S–7S.

Kleinman, R.E. and Walker, W.A. (1979). The enteromammary immune system: an important new concept in breast milk host defence. *Dig. Dis. Sci.* **24**, 876–82.

Bibliography

Kolars, J.C. *et al.* (1984). Yoghurt, an auto-digesting source of lactose. *New Engl. J. Med.* **310**, 1–3.

Koop, C.E. and Brannon, M.E. (1984). Breastfeeding: the community norm. Report of a workshop. *Public Health Rep.* **99**, (6) 550–8. [The full report is available from the National Center for Education in Maternal and Child Health, 3520 Prospect St. N.W., Washington, D.C. 20057, USA.]

Kumar, G.A., and Little, T.M. (1985). Has treatment for childhood gastroenteritis changed? *Br. med. J.* **290**, 1321–2. [This is a follow-up of the study discussed in 1981. (see Wharton 1981) The answer is that drugs are still given too much and oral rehydration too little.]

Kuroume, T. *et al.* (1976). Milk sensitivity and soy bean sensitivity in the production of eczematous manifestations in breastfed infants, with particular reference to intra-uterine sensitisation. *Ann. Allergy* **37**, 42–6.

La Luyer, B. *et al.* (1983). Ulcerative inflammatory colitis presenting as an allergy to bovine proteins: apropos of a neonatal case. *LARC Med.* (France) **3**, 206–209.

Lancet editorials:

(1981). Oral encounters with antigen. **i**, 702

(1981). Oral therapy for acute diarrhoea. **ii**, 615.

(1981). Coffee. **i**, 256.

(1982). Voluntary agreements do not halt epidemics. **ii**, 855.

(1983). Global ethics. **i**, 33.

(1983). 'Opren scandal' **i**, 219.

(1983). Meadow and Munchausen. **i**, 456.

(1983). Management of acute diarrhoea. **i**, 623–4.

(1983). Self-referral laboratories. **i**, 809; 989–90.

(1983). Colitis in term babies. **i**, 1083–4.

(1983). Childhood asthma. **ii**, 659–60; 790–2.

(1983). Inflammatory mediators of asthma **ii**, 829–30.

(1984). Adverse reactions to food. **i**, 900.

(1984). Infantile bloody diarrhoea and cows' milk allergy. **i**, 1159–60.

(1984). Prodomal itching in childhood asthma. **ii**, 154–5.

(1984). Do detergent residues damage the gut? **ii**, 384.

(1984). Complement C4 and drug-induced SLE. **ii**, 441–2.

Lappe, F.M. (1975). *Diet for a small planet.* Ballantine Books, New York. [The companion recipe book is Ewald, E.B. (1980) *Recipes for a small planet*, also published by Ballantine Books.]

Lawrence, R.A. (1985). *Breastfeeding: a guide for the medical profesion*, 2nd edn. C.V. Mosby, St. Louis. [Should be in multiple copies in medical libraries.]

Leach, P. (1981). *Baby and child.* Penguin, Harmondsworth. [For my money, still the best book on normal child development, although I think it is useless about allergy and unreliable about breast-feeding.]

—— (1979). *Who cares?* Penguin, Harmondsworth. [A passionate plea for the social and environmental changes that are needed to enable mothers to enjoy their under-threes.]

Lebenthal, E. (ed.) (1981). *Textbook of gastroenterology and nutrition in childhood*, 2 vols. Raven Press, New York. [Good basic text, though all

Food for thought

such books are out-of-date before they're printed.]
Lee, D.A. (1983). Prevalence and spectrum of asthma in childhood. *Br. med. J.* **286**, 1256–8.
Lessof, M. (ed.) (1983). *Clinical reactions to food.* Wiley, Chichester.
—— (1984). *Allergy.* Wiley, Chichester.
Lerman, S.J. *et al.* (1982). Treatment of giardiases: literature review and recommendations. *Clin. Pediatr.* **21**, 409–11.
Levinsky, R.J. (1981). Food antigen handling by the gut. *J. Trop. Pediatr.* **27**, 1–3.
Liard, R. *et al.* (1982). Wheezy bronchitis in infants and parents smoking habits. *Lancet* **i**, 334–5.
Lifschitz, F. (ed.) (1982). *Paediatric nutrition: infant feeding, deficiencies and diseases* Marcel Dekker, New York.
—— (1983). Delayed complete functional lactase activity sufficiency in breastfed infants. *J. Pediatr. Gastroent. Nutr.* **2**, 478–83.
Lindblad, B. and Rafter, J. (1980). Increased excretion of a brain depressor amine in infantile coeliac disease and in healthy infants on a high protein milk diet. *Acta Paediatr. Scand.* **69**, 643–6.
Little, C.H. *et al.* (1983). Platelet serotonin release in rheumatoid arthritis: a study in food-intolerant patients. *Lancet* **ii**, 297–9.
Littlewood, J.M. *et al.* (1980). Childhood coeliac disease is disappearing. (Letter.) *Lancet* **ii**, 1359.
Lloyd-Still, J.D. (1979). Chronic diarrhoea of childhood and the misuse of elimination diets. *J. Pediatr.* **95**, 10–3.
Lo, G.W. and Walker, W.A. (1982). Chronic protracted diarrhoea of infancy: a nutritional disease. *Pediatrics* **72**, 796–800.
Lothe, L., Lindberg, T. and Jakobsson, I. (1982). Cows' milk formula as a cause of infantile colic: a double-blind study. *Pediatrics* **70**, 7–10; letters, 299–300.
—— (1983). Cows' milk proteins cause colic in breastfed infants: a double-blind cross-over study. *Pediatrics* **71**, 268–71.
Lucas, A., McLaughlan, P. and Coombs, R.R.A. (1984). Latent anaphylactic sensitisation of infants of low birth weight to cows' milk proteins, *Br. med. J.* **289**, 1254–6.
Luoma, R. (1984). Environmental allergens and morbidity in atopic and non-atopic familes. *Acta Paediatr. Scand.* **73**, 448–53.
Macfarlane, P.I. and Miller, V. (1984). Human milk in the management of protracted diarrhea of infancy. *Arch. Dis. Child.* **59**, 260–3.
MacKarness, R. (1980). *Chemical victims.* Pan Books, London. [Anecdotal, controversial, and also extremely helpful to many people; without books such as this there may never have been such a rapid increase in research.]
McLaughlan, P. *et al.* (1981). Effect of heat on the anaphylactic-sensitising capacity of cows milk, goats milk and various infant formulae. *Arch. Dis. Child.* **56**, 165–71.
—— (1981). An oral screening procedure to determine the sensitising capacity of infant feeding formulae. *Clin. Allergy* **11**, 311–18.
—— (1983). Latent anaphylactic sensitivity of infants to cows' milk pro-

Bibliography

teins: histamine release from blood basophils. *Clin. Allergy* **13**, 1–9.

McLean, J. and Holmes, I. (1980). Transfer of anti-viral antibodies from mothers to their infants. *J. Clin. Microbiol.* **12**, 320–5.

—— (1980). Effect of antibodies, trypsin and trypsin inhibitors on susceptibility of neonates to rotavirus infection. *J. Clin. Microbiol.* **13**, 22–9.

Machtinger, S. *et al.* (1983). Infantile allergy and milk-specific antibodies in breast milk. (abstract). *J. Allergy Clin. Immunol.* **71**, 37.

Manning, D.J. *et al* (1985). Candida in mouth or on dummy? *Arch. Dis. Child.* **60**, 381–2. [44% of dummies were colonised with thrush!]

Manoff, R.K. and Cooke, T.M. (1980). Whose milk shall we market? *J. Trop. Pediatr.* **iii–iv**.

Martin, J. (1975). *Infant feeding 1975: attitudes and practices in England and Wales.* Her Majesty's Stationery Office (HMSO), London.

Martin, M.E. (1984). Serum complement changes during double-blind challenges in children with a history of food sensitivity. *Pediatrics* **73**, 532–7.

Mata, L. (1978). Breastfeeding: main promotor of infant health. *Am. J. Clin. Nutr.* **31**, 2058–65.

Matsamura, T. *et al.* (1967). Congenital sensitisation to food in humans. *Jpn. J. Allergy* **16**, 858.

Matthew, D. *et al.* (1977). Prevention of eczema *Lancet* **i**, 321.

May, C.D. *et al.* (1982). Immunologic consequences of feeding infants with cows milk and soy products. *Acta Paediatr. Scand.* **71**, 43–51.

—— (1985). Are confusion and controversy about food hypersensitivity really necessary? *J. Allergy Clin. Immunol.* **75**, 331–3.

Meadow, R. (1977). Munchausen syndrome by proxy: the hinterland of child abuse. *Lancet* **ii**, 343–5.

—— (1982). Munchausen syndrome by proxy. *Arch. Dis. Child.* **57**, 92–8.

—— (1985). Management of Munchausen syndrome by proxy. *Arch. Dis. Child.* **60**, 385–93.

Medawar, C. (1979). *Insult or injury? an enquiry into the marketing and advertising of British food and drug products in the Third World.* Social Audit, (9 Poland St London W1V 3DG).

Mellon, M. *et al.* (1983). No increase in cows' milk sensitisation after delayed ingestion in infancy. (abstract) *J. Allergy Clin. Immunol.* **71**, 37.

Meillon, R. and Reading, C. (1984). *Relatively speaking* Fontana, Australia. [The influence of genetics in pre-disposing us to particular diseases.]

Messenger, M. (1983). *The Breastfeeding book.* Century Publishing, London. [Beautifully set out, but uncritical of bottle-feeding, which all too often compounds the problem of the failure to thrive breast-fed infant. Also repeats and illustrates poor positioning techniques responsible for many difficulties. Otherwise sound enough generally.]

Metcalfe, D.D. and Kaliner, M.A. (1984). What is food to one . . . *New Engl. Med. J.* **345**, 399–400.

Michel, F.B. *et al.* (1980). Comparison of cord blood IgE concentrations and maternal allergy for the prediction of atopic diseases in infancy. *J. Allergy Clin. Immunol.* **65**, 422–30.

Food for thought

Miller, J.R. *et al.* (1983). The safety of egg-containing vaccines for egg-allergic patients. *Pediatrics* **71**, 568–73.

Milunsky, A. Friedman, E.A. and Gluck, L. (ed.) (1982). *Advances in perinatal medicine*, Vol. 2. Plenum Press, New York. [Chapter by Gaull, 'Human milk as food,' is essential reading.]

Minchin, M. (1984). Colic and other manifestations of food intolerance in normal breastfed infants and their families. *Proceedings*, 20th International Congress, International Confederation of Midwives, Sydney, September 1984.

—— (1985). *Breastfeeding matters*. George Allen and Unwin, Sydney/Alma Publications. [In this book I have developed mnay of the themes and controversies alluded to in the preceding pages, arguing that better motivation and management of breast-feeding are long overdue, and criticizing many long-cherished assumptions. Essential reading; first of a series to discuss infant feeding issues.]

Minford, A.M. *et al.* (1982). Food intolerance and food allergy in children. *Arch. Dis. Child.* **57**, 742–7.

Mitchell, E.B. *et al.* (1982). Inhaled allergens in infantile atopic eczema. *Lancet* **i**, 127; Letters, Feb. 27; Editorial, Oct. 9.

Monro, J. *et al.* (1984). Migraine is a food allergic disease. *Lancet* **ii**, 719–22.

Moore, J. *et al.* (1985). Why do people seek treatment by alternative medicine? *Br. Med. J.* **290**, 28–9.

Narayanan, I. *et al.* (1981). The value of human milk in the prevention of infection in high-risk LBW infants. *J. Pediatr.* **99**, 496–9.

—— (1984). Randomised controlled trial of effect of raw and Holder pasteurised human milk and of formula supplements on incidence of neonatal infection. *Lancet* **ii**, 1111–13.

Nathan-Hill, A. (1980). *Against the unsuspected enemy*. New Horizon; available from AAA: see p. 193. [The personal history of AAA's founder.]

Nayman, R. *et al.* (1979). Observations on the composition of milk-substitute products for treatment of inborn errors of amino-acid metabolism: comparisons with human milk. A proposal to rationalize nutrient content of treatment products. *Am. J. Clin. Nutr.* **32**, 1279–89. [Important paper which seems to have been largely ignored.]

Neville, M.C. and Niefert, M.R. (1984). *Lactation: physiology, nutrition and breastfeeding*. Plenum Press, New York. [Textbook for a fascinating inter-disciplinary graduate course. Basic for medical and nursing libraries.]

Newson, E. and Newson, J. (1968, 1970). *Patterns of infant care*. Penguin, Harmondsworth. [This, and the books that succeeded it, are basic library resources for anyone dealing with real families. They document life in roughly 600 families being followed from birth of the first child until that child gives birth. Parents would be better understood by professionals were this part of every family medicine programme.]

Oakley, A. (1984). *Taking it like a woman*. Random House, New York.

O'Connell, E.J. and Logan, G.B. (1974). Parental smoking in

Bibliography

childhood asthma. *Ann. Allergy* **32**, 172–5.

Ogra, S.S. *et al.* (1978). Immunologic aspects of human colostrum and milk: interaction with the intestinal immunity of the neonate. *Adv. Med. Biol.* **107**, 95–107.

Oski, F.A. (1983). *Don't drink your milk!* Beta Books, Sydney. [An American Professor of Pediatrics noted for his work on iron deficiency anemia argues strongly that milk can be harmful.]

—— (1983). Effect of iron therapy on behaviour performance in non-anemic iron-deficient infants. *Pediatrics* **71**, 877–80.

Packard, V. (1983). *Human milk and infant formula.* Academic Press, New York. [Entirely misleading, but fascinating book which manages to make formula sound safer than breast-feeding. The author, a dairy technologist, attempts to monopolize the middle ground of 'rationality' and objectivity: what he omits casts some doubts on such claims.]

Paganelli, R. *et al.* (1983). Differences between normal and milk-allergic subjects in their immune responses after milk ingestion. *Arch. Dis. Child.* **58**, 201–6.

Papageorgiou, N. *et al.* (1983). Neutrophil chemotactic activity in milk-induced asthma. *Pediatrics* **72**, 75.

Parihar, H. *et al.* (1984). The incidence of allergic diseases and feeding patterns in children up to 2 years of age. *Indian Pediatr. J.* **51**, 7–12.

Parke, A.L. and Hughes, G.R.V. (1981). Rheumatoid arthritis and food: a case study. *Br. med. J.* **282**, 2027–9.

Pearson, A.D.J. *et al.* (1982). Intestinal permeability in children with Crohn's disease and coeliac disease. *Br. med. J.* **285**, 20–1.

—— (1983). Food allergy: how much in the mind? *Lancet* **i**, 1259–61; Letters, **ii**, 45; critique, Hunter (1984). 'Sub-optimal technique' explains the discrepancy between this and other studies, but it is widely quoted by those who persist in believing that most patients are neurotic.

Peatfield, R.C. *et al.* (1984). The prevalence of diet-induced migraine. *Cephalalgia* **4**, 179–83.

Persico, M. *et al.* (1983). Recurrent middle ear infections in infants: the protective role of maternal breastfeeding. *Ear Nose Throat J.* **62**, 20–4, 26–7, 31.

Philbrick, H. and Philbrick, J. (1974). *The bug book: harmless insect controls.* Garden Way Publishing, Vermont. [For chemical-sensitive gardeners.]

Philpott, W.H. and Kalita, D.K. (1980). *Brain Allergies: the psycho-nutrient connection.* Keats Publishing Co, New Canaan, Connecticut. [When I first read this it seemed way out. Since then much more has emerged within orthodox medicine about central nervous system effects of foods. Worth reading and considering.]

Pittard, W.B. (1981). Special properties of human milk. *Birth and the Family J.* **8**, 229–35.

Platt-Mills, T. *et al.* (1982). Reduction of bronchial hyper-reactivity during prolonged antigen avoidance. *Lancet* **ii**, 675–7.

Podell, R.N. (1983). Intracutaneous and sublingual provocation and neutralization. *Clinical Ecology* **II**, 13–20.

Food for thought

Poland, R.L. (1981). Breast milk jaundice. *J. Pediatr.* **99**, 86–7.

Population Report LI (1979). *Tobacco: hazards to human health and reproduction.* Available from the Population Information Program, Johns Hopkins University, Baltimore.

Price, A. and Bamford, N. (1983). *The breastfeeding guide for the working woman.* Simon and Schuster, New York.

Rao, A.R. (1977). Human breast milk as commercial infant food. *J. Trop. Pediatr. Environ. Child Health*, **23**, 286–8.

Raphael, D. (1985). *Only mothers know.* Greenwood Press, Connecticut. [A sad and rather silly book, I think , which needs detailed criticism to expose its biases and assumptions. Will be reviewed in later work.]

Rapp, D. (1980). *Allergies and your family.* Sterling Publishing, New York.

—— (1979). *Allergies and the hyperactive child.* Simon and Schuster, New York. [Excellent basic books, recommended for group libraries.]

Rea, W.J. (1981). Recurrent environmentally triggered thrombophlebitis: a five-year follow-up. *Ann. Allergy* **47**, 338–44.

—— (1984). Elimination of oral food challenge reaction by injection of food extracts: a double-blind evaluation. *Arch. Otolaryngol.* **110**, 248–52.

Reeves, W.G. (1983). Development of clinical immunology and allergy in the U.K.: common problems and solutions. *Lancet* **ii**, 721–3.

Rhodes, J.M. *et al.* (1984). Colonic Crohn's disease and use of oral contraception. *Br. med. J.* **288**, 595–6.

Rippere, V. (1983). *The allergy problem.* Thorsons Publishers, Wellingborough. [A book about the problems allergy victims face after diagnosis, many of which are socially created and hence remediable. Recommended for general reading, particularly by those who think this is merely another fad.]

Roberts, S.A. and Soothill, J.F. (1982). Provocation of allergic response by supplementary feeds of cows' milk. *Arch. Dis. Child.* **57**, 127–30.

Rodgers, B. (1978). Infant feeding and later ability and attainment: a longitudinal study. *Develop. Med. Child Neurol.* **20**, 421–6.

Rosenhall, L. (1982). Evaluation of intolerance to analgesics, preservatives and food colorants with challenge tests. *Eur. J. Resp. Dis.* **63**, 410.

Royal College of Physicians and British Nutrition Foundation Joint Report: food intolerance and food aversion. *J. R. Coll. Phys. London* **78**. [Available from the College at 11 St. Andrew's Place, Regent's Park, NW1 4LE, England, £3 posted.]

Ruokonen, J. *et al.* (1982). Elimination diets in the treatment of secretory otitis media. *Int. J. Pediatr. Otorhinolaryngol.* **4**, 39–46.

Russell, G. (1983). *A practical guide for fathers.* Sphere, London. [Since allergic children can be very demanding, fathers must be involved if the marriage is to survive. This is a good general guide to useful involvement.]

Saarinen, U. (1979). Prolonged breastfeeding as prophylaxis for allergic disease. *Lancet* **ii**, 163–6.

Bibliography

—— (1982). Prolonged breastfeeding as prophylaxis for recurrent otitis media. *Acta Paediatr. Scand.* **71**, 567–71.

Sage, D. (1981). Intradermal drug testing following anaphylactoid reactions during anaesthesia. *Anaesth. intens. Care* **9**, 381.

Said, G. *et al.* (1984). Infantile colic and parental smoking. *Br. med. J.* **289**, 660.

Salisbury, L. and Blackwell, A.G. (1981). *An Administrative Petition to the U.S. Food and Drug Administration and Department of Health and Human Services, to alleviate domestic infant formula misuse and to provide informed infant feeding choice.* Available from Public Advocates. Inc., 1535 Mission St., San Francisco, CA. 94103, USA.

Salter, E. (1983). *Child of nine: feeding with love and good sense.* Bull Publishing Co., Palo Alto, CA. [Detailed dietetic advice; not allergy.]

Sampson, A.A. (1983). Role of immediate food hypersensitivity in the pathogenesis of atopic dermatitis. *J. Allergy Clin. Immunol.* **71**, 473–80.

Schwartz, H.J. (1983). Sensitivity to ingested metalbisulphite. *J. Allergy Clin. Immunol.* **71**, 487–9.

Second International Symposium on Immunological and Clinical Problems of Food Allergy, Milan, 1982. *Ann. Allergy* (1983) **51**, 2 part 2, 218–328.

Shambaugh, G.E. and Weil, R.J. (1980). The diagnosis and evaluation of allergic disorders with food intolerance in Menier's disease. *Otolaryngol. Clin. N. Am.* **13**, 671–9.

—— (1984). Allergic therapy for Menier's disease. *Am. J. Otol.* **5**, 556–7.

Shenassa, M. and Gerrard, J.W. (1984). Cow's milk allergy developing when breast-feeding stops. *Clinical Ecology* **1**, 72–4.

Shinwell, E. and Gorodischer, R. (1982). Totally vegetarian diets and infant nutrition. *Pediatrics* **70**, 582–6.

Shmerling, D.H. (1983). Dietary protein induced colitis in breastfed infants. *J. Pediatr.* **102**, 500.

Simoons, F.J. (1978). Lactose intolerance. *Digestive Diseases* **23**, 963.

Smith, L. (1980). *The encyclopedia of baby and child care.* Warner Books, New York. [Interesting contrast with Jolly in amount of medical information given to parents.]

Smithells, R.W. *et al.* (1983). Further experience of vitamin supplementation for prevention of NTD recurrences. *Lancet* **i**, 1027–31. [See also *Lancet* (2982) **ii**, 1255–6; (1983) **ii**, 798–9.]

Soothill, J.F., Hayward, A.R., and Wood, C.B.S. (1983). *Paediatric immunology.* Blackwell Scientific Publications, Oxford. [Essential reading for professionals and especially for those who believe early infant feeding is of little significance and complementary feedings of cows' milk acceptable.]

—— (1979). Food allergy. *J. Maternal Child Health*, 385–9.

—— (1984). Prevention of food allergic disease. *Ann. Allergy*, **53**, (6 Pt. 2) 689–91. [This issue contains many other articles of interest.]

Speer, F. and Dockhorn, R. (ed.) (1975). *Allergy and immunology in childhood.* C.C. Thomas, Illinois. [Although out-of-date in some

Food for thought

respects, this contains a wealth of clinical observation that time continued to validate.]

Stables, J. (1981). *A mother's guide to breastfeeding.* Star Books. [Available from the Association of Breastfeeding Mothers, see p. 198. Simple basic book; like all such, needing to be supplemented with more specialist literature.]

Stanway, P. and Stanway, A. (1983). *Breast is best.* Pan Books, London. [The most comprehensive and reliable basic book on breast-feeding cheaply available. Sheila Kitzinger's *The experience of breastfeeding* is better on some emotional aspects, but for sound up-to-date information Stanways remain the best choice. Their various babycare books are also excellent, as is *The breast* (Granada, London, 1982). This is the only book about women's breasts to include consideration of their reproductive significance.]

Stare, F. (1980). Diet and hyperactivity: is there a relationship? *Pediatrics* **66**, 521. (Letters, **67**, 913, 937; **68**, 300–1; **69**, 128; 250.)

Stuart, C.A. *et al.* (1984). Passage of cows' milk protein in breast milk. *Clin Allergy* **14**, 533–5.

Svedlund, J. *et al.* (1983). Controlled trial of psychotherapy in irritable bowel syndrome. *Lancet* **ii**, 589–91. [Often misread as disproving dietary etiology, when reduction in stress levels may merely have improved patient tolerance levels.]

Swinson, C. *et al.* (1983). Coeliac disease and malignancy. *Lancet* **i**, 111–15.

Taitz, L.S. (1983). Soy feeding in infancy. *Arch. Dis. Child.* **57**, 814–15.

—— and Armitage, B.L. (1984) Goats' milk for infants and children. *Br. med. J.* **288**, 428–9.

Tallerman, K.H. (1934). Sensitivity to cows' milk proteins in acute gastroenteritis. *Arch. Dis. Child.* **IX**, 189–93.

Tanner, M.S. and Stocks, R.J. (1984). *Neonatal gastroenterology: contemporary issues.* Intercept, Newcastle on Tyne.

Task Force on the Assessment of the Scientific Evidence Relating to Infant Feeding Practices and Infant Health (1984). Report. *Pediatrics*, **74**, 4, 2. Suppl. [This is very patchy indeed: quality of chapters ranges from excellent to dreadful, with an obvious bias towards reassuring people that infant formula is as safe as breast milk. Will be reviewed in greater detail in a later volume of my new series, *Breastfeeding matters.*]

Taubman, B. (1984). Clinical trial of the treatment of colic by modification of parent–infant interaction. *Pediatrics*, **74**, 998–1003. [Teaching parents to respond to their babies cries humanely resulted (as could be expected) in decreased crying. This neither disproves nor proves the food intolerance link in any case!]

Tay, J.T. and Wong, H.B. (1980). Cows' milk intolerance in Singapore. *Mod. Med. Asia.* **16**, 28–34.

Taylor, E. (1984). Diet and behaviour. *Arch. Dis. Child.* **59**, 97–8.

Taylor, R.H. (1982). Clinical tests for hypolactasia, lactose malabsorption, and lactose intolerance. *Lancet* **ii**, 766.

Bibliography

Thames Television/The Mental Health Foundation. (1982). *Someone to talk to: a directory of self-help and support services in the community.* [Available from 8 Hallam St., London, W1N 6DH.]

Thomas, D.B. (1981). Aetiological associations in infantile colic: an hypothesis. *Aust. Paediatr. J.* **17**, 292–5.

Tinkelman, D.G. and Bock, S.A. (1984). Anaphylaxis presumed to be caused by beef containing streptomycin. *Ann. Allergy* **53**, 283–4.

Tipton, W.R. (1983). Evaluation of skin tests in the diagnosis of IgE mediated disease. *Pediatr. Clin. N. Am.* **30**, 785–94.

Tomasi, T.B. *et al.* (1980). Mucosal immunity: the origin and migration patterns of cells in the secretory system. *J. Allergy Clin. Immunol.* **65**, 12–19.

Tripp, J.H. and Candy, D.C. (1984). Oral rehydration fluids. *Arch. Dis. Child.* **59**, 99–101.

Twarog, F.J. (1983). Urticaria in childhood. *Ped. Clin. N. Am.* **30**, 837–48.

Udall, J.N. (1982). Dietary proteins, serum immunoglobulins, and antigens. *J. Pediatr. Gastroent. Nutr.* **1**, 155–6.

Underwood, B.A. and Hofvander, Y. (1982). Appropriate timing for complementary feeding of the breastfed infant. *Acta. Pediatr. Scand.*, Suppl. 294. [Essential reading on this subject.]

Valman, H. (1979). Infant feeding and feeding problems. *Br. med. J.* **280**, 458.

Van Asperen, P.P. *et al.* (1983). Immediate food hypersensitivity reactions on the first known exposure to the food. *Arch. Dis. Child.* **58**, 253–6.

—— (1983). Experience with an elimination diet in children with atopic dermatitis. *Clin. Allergy* **13**, 479–85.

Van Metre, (1983). Critique of controversial and unproven procedures for diagnosis and therapy of allergic disorders. *Ped. Clin. N. Am.* **30**, 5 807–18.

Ventura, A. *et al.* (1981). Reaginic hypersensitivity to cows' milk proteins *Helv. Pediatr. Acta* **36**, 237–40.

Verkasalo, M. *et al.* (1981). Changing patterns of cows' milk intolerance. *Acta Paediatr. Scand.* **70**, 289–95.

Vittoria, J.C. *et al.* (1982). Enteropathy related to fish, rice and chicken. *Arch. Dis. Child.* **57**, 44–8.

Von Witt, V. (1978). Chronic illness and hidden food allergies. *Mod. Med. (UK)* July, pp. 8–14.

Walker, W.A. (1975). Antigen absorption from the small intestine and gastrointestinal disease. *Pediatr. Clin. N. Am.* **22**, 731–46.

—— and Block, K.J. (1983). Gastrointestinal transport of macromolecules in the pathogenesis of food allergy. *Ann. Allergy* **51**, 2 pt. 2., 240–5.

Walther, F.J. and Kootstra, G. (1983). Necrotizing enterocolitis as a result of cows' milk allergy? *Z. Kinderchir.* **38**, 110–11.

Warnasuriya, N. *et al.* (1980). Atopy in parents of children dying with SIDS. *Arch. Dis. Child.* **55**, 879–82.

Food for thought

Warner, J.O. (1980). Food allergy in full breastfed infants. *Clin. Allergy* **10**, 133–6.

—— and Hathaway, M.J. (1984). Allergic form of Meadow's syndrome (Munchausen by proxy.) *Arch. Dis. Child.* **59**, 151–6.

Weissbluth, M. (1984). Treatment of infantile colic with dicyclomine hydrochloride. *J. Pediatr.* **104**, 951–5.

Wells, D. (1983). *What shall I give him today?* [50 milk, egg and additive-free recipes. Simple but useful. Available for 85p. posted from R.A. and H.D. Wells, 19a Parton Rd., Churchdown, Gloucester GL3 2AB.]

Werner, D. (1980). *Where there is no doctor: a village health care handbook.* Macmillan Tropical Community Health Manuals, London. [Low-cost, high-quality, easily-understood primary health care manual that has more uses in affluent societies than is often realized. Worth having in every library.]

Wessel, M.A. *et al.* (1954). Paroxysmal fussing in infancy, sometimes called colic. *Pediatrics* **14**, 42–54.

Wharton, B.A. (1981). Gastroenteritis in Britain—management at home. *Br. med. J.* **282**, 1277. [In the same issue, p. 1300, there is a disturbing survey of the usual treatment of gastroenteritis in 181 children. Education about oral rehydration is long overdue in affluent societies. Up-dated, Kumar (1985).]

Whitfield, R. *et al.* (1981). Validity of routine clinical test weighing as a measure of the intake of breastfed babies. *Arch. Dis. Child.* **56**, 919–21.

Wilkinson, A.W. (ed.) (1981). *The immunology of infant feeding.* Plenum Press, New York. [Discusses issues such as the immunological implications of donated breast milk and artificial formulae. Still worth reading.]

Williams, R. and Kalita, D. (1977). *A physician's guide to orthomolecular medicine.* Pergamon Press, New York.

Winick, M. (ed.) (1979). *Human nutrition: a comprehensive treatise.* Vol. 1 *Nutrition: pre and post-natal development.* Plenum Press, New York.

Winter, R.A. (1978). *A consumer's dictionary of food additives.* Crown Publishers, New York. [Very informative, but not reassuring!]

Wood, C.B.S. and Walker-Smith, J.A. (1981). *MacKeith's infant feeding and feeding difficulties.* Churchill Livingstone, Edinburgh. [Extremely useful book which combines some of the clinical skills of the past with only slightly out-of-date information. One of the best infant feeding texts.]

Workman, E., Hunter, J. and Alun Jones, V. (1984). *The allergy diet: how to overcome your food intolerance.* Methuen Positive Health Guide series, Sydney/London. [The recipe book you can happily take to your doctor!]

World Health Organization, (1982). *Women and breastfeeding.* WHO, 1211 Geneve 27, Switzerland.

Wray, D. *et al.* (1982). Food allergens and basal histamine release in recurrent apthous stomatitis. *Oral Surg.* **54**, 388–95.

Bibliography

Wright, S. and Burton, J.L. (1982). Oral evening primrose seed oil improves atopic eczema. *Lancet* **ii**, 1120–2.

Wright, W.C. *et al.* (1975). Decreased bactericidal activity of leukocytes of stressed newborn infants. *Pediatrics* **56**, 398–403.

Woodruff, C. (1983). Breastfeeding or infant formula should be continued for 12 months. (Letter.) *Pediatrics* **71**, 984–5.

Youlten, L.J.F. (1983). Investigation of acute adverse reactions to intravenous anaesthetics. Paper given at British Society for Allergy and Clinical Immunology meeting, London, November, 1983.

Yoshiaka, H. *et al.* (1983). Developmental differences of intestinal flora in the neonatal period in breastfed and bottlefed infants. *Pediatrics* **72**, 317.

Zernov, N.G. *et al.* (1983). Chronic esophagitis in food allergy in children. *Pediatriia* (USSR) **9**, 68–9.

Zoppi, G. *et al.* (1983). Diet and antibody response to vaccinations in healthy infants. *Lancet* **ii**, 11–13. (Letters, **ii**, 341–2; 861.)

Artifical feeding carries risks. Infants who are fed artifically are biologically different from those who are breast-fed. Their blood carries different patterns of amino acids, some of which may be at levels high enough to cause anxiety. The composition of their body fat is different. They are fed a variety of carbohydrates to which no other mammalian offspring is exposed in neonatal life. They have higher plasma osmolality, urea, and electrolyte levels. Their guts are colonised by a potentially invasive type of microflora, at the same time as they are exposed to large amounts of foreign protein resulting in an immunologic response. In addition, they are deprived of the various immune factors present in human milk. All these factors need to be taken into consideration every time a decision is made not to breastfeed an infant, for inherent in such a decision are known and unknown risks to the infant. Certainly, in those instances where the physiologic reserves of the infant are low, or have been compromised as in pre-term babies, those who have suffered hypoxia, in cases of major surgery and in stresses of all forms, feeding with the mother's milk should be considered obligatory.

G.J. Ebrahim, *Breastfeeding, the biological option* pp. 59–60,
Macmillan (1978).

Notes

CHAPTER 1 FOOD INTOLERANCE

1. cf. Reeves (1983). I agree entirely that 'Separation of some immunological disorders, for example those of an atopic nature, from the rest is both contrived and arbitrary, and will not advance our understanding of disorders characterised by an immunological response to environmental immunogens.'
2. A simple summary can be found in Eagle (1979), pp. 198–204; also Gerrard (1980).
3. Berman and MacDonnell (1981). Chapter 1.
4. Chemicals are thought to be haptens, that is, they are not antigens until they combine with a body protein. After that they can stimulate an immune response. (They can also affect the body in other ways, such as affecting enzyme pathways.) Technical distinctions are not important for our purposes, the term 'excitant' is used to mean what parents mean when they talk of allergens: that is, anything that causes a reaction.
5. Histamine causes blood-vessel dilation and increased permeability, as well as smooth muscle contraction. 'This in part causes wheezing and colic.' Forsythe (1977), p. 4.
6. Forsythe (1977). p. 6. Fever does NOT mean that infection is necessarily present, as many mothers who have treated mastitis are aware.
7. Soothill (1979). In actual practice allergy and intolerance frequently co-exist in the same person.
8. Simoons (1978); Taylor (1982). Because a majority of people are lactose-intolerant after infancy, the indiscriminate advertising and promotion of milk, and its use as a relief food, have been questioned. Was the huge campaign aimed at teenagers a factor in the rising asthma death rate, I wonder?
9. Many women routinely consume the equivalent of two or more litres of milk daily, although the recommended amounts are much less, cf. p. 00. This is a new food belief: only a generation or two back, milk was regarded with suspicion, cf. Murcott (1983).
10. The effect of different milks on gut bacteria is discussed in Stanway (1978); Wilkinson (1981); and Soothill, Hayward, and Wood (1983). Soothill states categorically that for this and other reasons, 'early artificial feeding, including supplements, should never be done unnecessarily', p. 116.
11. Discussed at greater length in my forthcoming book, *Breastfeeding matters*.
12. Bullen and Willis (1971).

Notes: Chapters 1–2

CHAPTER 2 EFFECTS AND VICTIMS OF FOOD
INTOLERANCE

1. Whose babies are to be the guinea-pigs in trials of formulae that 'need
   not mirror breast milk'? Dugdale (1981) argues that it is 'unlikely
   that breast milk (would) maintain optimal growth of body and particularly of the brain' as the mother must survive too. The idea that
   scientists could do better does not accord well with the record to date,
   cf. Minchin (1985). As Gaull (1982) stated, 'It is conceivable that a
   departure from it (human milk) may represent nutritional improvement, but how to establish that this is a real improvement without a
   later price to pay is a major scientific problem.' Soothill again sum-
   med it up neatly: 'The pressing need to prevent the spread of
   unnecessarily artificial feeding in developing countries should not
   deflect us from awareness of our profound ignorance of the effects
   such changes may have had in developed countries. Immunological
   theory can suggest that many adverse effects, early and late, may
   arise from the deprivation or inactivation of maternal protective systems, perhaps especially in some vulnerable individuals. *The only
   rational deduction is that such a physiological system should be left
   undisturbed, unless unavoidable, until we know for certain that it is
   safe to do so,*' (my emphasis).
2. Individual needs can also vary significantly: cf Winick (1981), p. 446.
3. Jelliffe and Jelliffe (eds.) (1982), p. 50.
4. Isbister (1979), pp. 74–5.
5. Lerman and Walker (1982), p. 409; Harries (1979), p. 1101.
6. Gillin (1983).
7. Crook (1983).
8. The implications of our changed nutritional habits for less developed
   countries has been and is horrendous. It is obscene for food to be
   used as a political weapon; for stock to be fattened on grain needed
   by people; for the seas to be devastated to provide high quality pet
   food while millions of children starve; for infant mortality and morbidity from hunger to be rising in the world's richest countries. Support for UNICEF's child revolution and work to improve maternal
   health should come from those of us fortunate enough to have well-
   fed children.
9. cf. papers by Ogra, Carlsson, Walker, Suskind, Soothill, and others in
   Freier and Eidelman (1981).
10. Enzymes (and hormones and mitogens and much else) in human milk
    have been poorly studied as yet. Note the changing nature of breast
    milk compared with an inflexible formula.
11. Walker (1975).
12. This applies also to respiratory allergens, cf. Warner (1983).
13. *Food intolerance and food aversion. Joint report of the Royal College
    of Physicians and the British Nutrition Foundation* (hereafter
    RCP/BNF Report) (1984) p. 13, cf. also Matsamura *et al.* (1967);
    Kuroume *et al.* (1976).

14. But the child of the non-atopic family may not develop immediately the type and severity of symptom that is unmistakably allergic or intolerant. Until recently, few looked for the other end of what must be a normal distribution curve: the less dramatic, sub-clinical symptoms such as colic, which may indeed be 'normal' in our society because our normal treatment of infants has included hyperallergenic exposure neonatally.
15. DHSS (1980).
16. Lawrence (1985).
17. Papers by Leefsma, Naylor, Verronen, and others in Freier and Eidelman (1981).

CHAPTER 3   GENERAL SYMPTOMS

1. Rapp (1978), pp. 8–10.
2. RCP/BNF Report, p. 8.
3. Kidd (1983).
4. Cant *et al.* (1984).
5. RCP/BNF Report, p. 8.
6. Behavioural problems are increasingly recognized as being related to food intolerance problems, though in a more complex manner than was originally proposed by Feingold supporters, cf. Gerrard (1980); Egger *et al.* (1985).
7. Hill (1981).
8. Not enough work has been done to ascertain whether very young infants being fully breast-fed have the capacity for complete recovery of intestinal function once the mother eliminates the antigen from her diet. Since breast milk contains growth factors specific for intestinal development, this is possible. But many children do retain a degree of sensitivity indefinitely.
9. 'About children', Australian Broadcasting Commission radio broadcast, 4 January, 1983.
10. In Australia estimates are that one in seven suffers major allergic disease. In the USA 20 per cent are allergic by the age of 20; one third of all chronic conditions are due to allergy; one third of all school absences are due to asthma (Lawrence, 1980 edition, p. 249).
11. Rippere (1983) discusses the impact on the family and individual.
12. Mackarness (1980), p. 46.
13. Dr. Mavis Gunther made this point in correspondence.
14. For discussion of the complexities of digestion, see Chandra (1984); Tanner and Stocks (1984), or Lebenthal (1982). If an allergic reaction causes damage to the gut lining other enzymes in that lining may be unable to break down other foods, and so secondary intolerances develop. In some breast-fed babies, high stool levels of lactose follow exposure to certain excitants in mother's milk; only finding the allergen will stop the lactose intolerance. This also works the other way: being born with minor defects in pancreas or gall

bladder, or with lower than normal enzyme levels, could allow undigested food by-products to damage the gut; a damaged gut more readily becomes sensitive to allergens.
15. Foresight (1980).
16. Walker (1975).
17. The comparison with drug addition is apt. Mackarness now works with chemically addicted patients, using the same methods as with foods.
18. Rapp (1978), p. 57.

CHAPTER 4 FOOD INTOLERANCE IN INFANCY

1. Dugdale (1981).
2. Lawrence (1980 edition) p. 14; Edmeades *et al.* (1982); Cunningham in Jelliffe and Jelliffe, *Advances* Vol. 1. (1981); (1984).
3. Media images of babies promote the concept of them as either immaculate and angelic, or miserable and crying, with the latter image predominant. Yet my children (and I) become distressed by the very sound, which they recognize as a call for help.
4. Doctors who have worked in less developed countries frequently comment that colic is virtually unknown there.
5. Ford (1982).
6. Lothe *et al.* (1982).
7. RCP/BNF Report, p. 15.
8. Jakobsson and Lindberg (1978).
9. Jakobsson and Lindberg (1979).
10. Lothe *et al.* (1982).
11. Jakobsson and Lindberg (1983).
12. Gerrard (1979).
13. Hemmings (1981); Curtis-Jenkins (1981).
14. Evans *et al.* (1981).
15. Drawn from a number of sources, but checked against maternal experience here in Australia.
16. Harrison *et al.* (1976).
17. Ebrahim (1978) provides an excellent outline for investigation of the growth-retarded infant.
18. Firer *et al.* (1981). This study did not examine neonatal feeding, maternal diet, or maternal allergic history before making conclusions about 'exclusively' breast-fed children.
19. Articles by Bullen and Wharton in Wilkinson (1981); Cunningham in Jelliffe and Jelliffe (1981).
20. Gerrard (1983).
21. Gerrard (1983).
22. Buisseret (1982).
23. Taurine has been almost totally absent from infant formula for 100 years because it was not known to be essential. After years of debate it was added in 1984, and the companies are using its presence as a major advertising feature!

Food for thought

24. For the worst possible case against human milk and an amazingly rosy view of formula, all done in the most 'objective' style, read Packard (1983). The author is a dairy technologist.
25. Soothill (1983), p. 120.
26. A notable recent case was Kahlia Chamberlain, whose mother was forced to leave her at five months of age after Lindy's (in my view wrongful) conviction for the murder of her previous child, Azaria, was upheld. After Kahlia failed to thrive on the bottle, another Adventist mother weaned her 10 month-old baby to feed Kahlia, who accepted wet-nursing as happily as any baby in another society. It is interesting to speculate as to whether the incredible stress to which Lindy was subjected during pregnancy was relevant to Kahlia's intolerance of milk.
27. Glaxo, in the early 1920s, was 'not only perfect from a scientific and clinical point of view, but . . . so easily prepared that even in the hands of the most ignorant or careless person, . . . infants would thrive.' So said a medical officer of health; he was doubtless believed because government clinics dispensed it by the ton.
28. Campbell (1981).
29. Jelliffe and Jelliffe, *Adverse effects* . . . (1982), pp. 575–89.
30. Ebrahim (1978).
31. Rao (1977).
32. Hambraeus (1977).
33. *Assignment children* (1981), pp. 139–67.
34. Price and Bamford (1983).
35. cf. World Health Organisation's pamphlet, *Women and breastfeeding* for a brief overview of necessary changes.
36. ICM (International Confederation of Midwives) (1984).
37. Oakley (1984), p. 87.
38. Von Witt (1978).
39. There are very few circumstances where supplementation of the breast-fed baby is anything but harmful. Dark-skinned mothers living in polluted or cold climates may need vitamin D supplementation; cultural habits may accentuate that need. But in general supplementation of the mother is preferable to supplementation of the baby.
40. Some of the earlier trials funded by the food industry can now be seen as severely defective in methodology (for example, using chocolate as the placebo!) Feingold never disputed that chemically-sensitive children might not also be milk- sugar- and chocolate-sensitive: much later work is proving him right to suspect that food additives are an additional and for the most part unnecessary problem.
41. *Pediatrics* (1982), 69 (2) A9.
42. Littlewood *et al.* (1980); Challacombe and Baylis (1980).
43. Gruskay (1982); May *et al.* (1982).
44. Atherton, in Fisons *Second workshop* (1983), p. 143, stated that 'the use of so-called control diets rich in soy milk (which contains a

relatively large amount of essential fatty acids) may need to be re-assessed.'
45. McLaughlan (1981).
46. RCP/BNF Report, p. 13.

CHAPTER 5 INHALANT PROBLEMS

1. Rubinfeld (1982).
2. Population Report LI (1979), *Tobacco, hazards to human health and reproduction.*
3. Cunningham (1981), pp. 156–7.
4. Evans (1979).
5. Jelliffe and Jelliffe (1982). *Adverse Effects* . . . pp. 129–34.
6. Correspondence with Dr. P. Hartmann, Biochemistry Department, University of Western Australia, Perth.
7. O'Connell (1974) concluded that 'parents must recognise that it is necessary to choose in some instances between their own pleasure and their child's health.'
8. *Population Report LI* (1979); *Lancet* editorial (1982) **ii**, 855.

CHAPTER 6 MEDICAL TREATMENTS

1. Chunn (1981); van Metre (1983); Tipton (1983).
2. cf. the current debate over whether women at risk for neural tube defects should be assigned to a randomized controlled trial in which some would receive peri-conceptual vitamins and others placebo. Surely women should be well-represented in any such decision-making debates.
3. *Lancet* (1982) **ii**, 919; 1050–1.
4. Jakobsson and Lindberg (1978).
5. Egger *et al.* (1983).
6. Rippere (1983).
7. Williams and Kalita (1977). Other reading available from the Canadian Schizophrenia Foundation.
8. Meadow (1982).
9. Meadow (1977).
10. Meadow (1977), p. 97.
11. *Lancet* editorial, (1983) **i**, 456.
12. Meadow (1982), p. 97.
13. Warner and Hathaway (1984).
14. Warner and Hathaway, p. 151.
15. RCP/BNF Report, p. 37.
16. Warner and Hathaway (1984), p. 154.
17. Warner and Hathaway (1984).
18. Meadow (1982, p. 95.

Food for thought

19. Warner and Hathaway (1984), p. 155.
20. Smith (1980).
21. Jolly (1977).
22. RCP/BNF Report, p. 15.
23. Forman (1980).

CHAPTER 7 FOOD INTOLERANCE AND THE FAMILY

1. Crook (1975).
2. This advice is now routine; however patients need to be aware of their own capabilities. cf. Rubinfeld (1982), pp. 30–1.
3. Wright (1975).
4. Johnstone *et al.* (1975).
5. Wright and Burton (1982).
6. Graham (1981). Other material available from HACSG (see p. 00).
7. RCP/BNF Report, p. 14.
8. World health bodies have recommended the following order of priorities for failed lactation in developing countries: Re-establishment of lactation; breast-feeding by surrogate; feeding non-human milk as a milk product; feeding a cereal/other staple gruel augmented by milk/other protein sources.
9. Rea, in Gerrard (1980).
10. *Breastfeeding Abstrats* (1982) **1**, (4).
11. RCP/BNF Report, p. 19.

CHAPTER 8 DRUGS AND THEIR ACTION

1. Youlten (1983).

CHAPTER 9 SOME UNANSWERED QUESTIONS

1. Speer and Dockhorn (1973), p. 403.
2. Speer and Dockhorn (1973), p. 2.

CHAPTER 11 WHAT TO DO IN PREGNANCY AND LACTATION

1. Eaton (1982), p. 18.
2. Johnstone (1981).
3. Hamburger (1983).
4. Matthew *et al.* (1977).

CHAPTER 12 HOW TO SUCCEED AT EXCLUSIVE BREAST-FEEDING

1. Lawrence (1980 edition), p. 176.
2. Valman (1980).
3. Whitfield *et al.* (1981).

Notes: Chapters 6–23

CHAPTER 14 BUT I'M BOTTLE-FEEDING: WHAT CAN I DO?

1. Gibson and Kneebone (1981).
2. Lothe *et al.* (1982).
3. Seminar on cows' milk intolerance, November 1982. Royal Children's Hospital, Parkville, Victoria 3052. Proceedings available.

CHAPTER 15 INTRODUCING OTHER FOODS TO THE INTOLERANT BABY

1. Underwood and Hofvander (1982) remains the best overall discussion of the weaning dilemma. Some later symposia seem less objective.
2. Lawrence, (1980 edition) 311–12. Seeing the baby suckle, and knowing what to look for, are essential; most professionals are not trained in this area. Hence the development of a new specialty, the Lactation Consultant. More detail in *Breastfeeding matters* (in press).
3. Rapp (1980), pp. 80–4.

CHAPTER 16 HOME MANAGEMENT OF DIARRHOEAL DISEASE

1. *Lancet* (1983) **i**, 55.
2. Jelliffe and Jelliffe (1981) *Advances* . . . p. v.

CHAPTER 17 HOME TESTING FOR FOOD INTOLERANCE

1. *Ann. Allergy* (1979) **40** (6) 393.
2. RCP/BNF Report, p. 9.
3. RCP/BNF Report, p. 36.
4. RCP/BNF Report, p. 9.
5. Lloyd-Still (1979).

CHAPTER 20 SOME CHANGES TO WORK FOR

1. Hamburger (1983).

CHAPTER 23 THE JOINT REPORT OF THE ROYAL COLLEGE OF PHYSICIANS AND BRITISH NUTRITION FOUNDATION

1. RCP/BNF Report, pp. 20–3.
2. RCP/BNF Report, p. 21.
3. Pearson *et al.* (1983).

Food for thought

4. Egger *et al.* (1983).
5. Svedlund *et al.* (1983).
6. All professionals should read Rippere (1983).
7. RCP/BNF Report, p. 21.
8. RCP/BNF Report, p. 36.
9. RCP/BNF Report, p. 15, 21.
10. Marital problems were common among families receiving inadequate medical help; in some cases undiagnosed illness in children caused divorce. There is a tendency to see marital breakdown as proof of psychological disorders in the mothers, which explained their children's problems. Despite the high marital breakdown rates among doctors, the clear implication in some writing is that the fact of being a single parent is evidence of maternal instability.
11. RCP/BNF Report, p. 22.
12. In neither Australia nor the UK does the amount of money spent seem to bear any relationship to the degree of patient satisfaction with advice given, if my correspondents are a representative sample. Rather, patient satisfaction depends on whether their perceived problems are better after following the advice given.
13. RCP/BNF Report, p. 7.
14. RCP/BNF Report, p. 12.
15. RCP/BNF Report, p. 15.
16. Kajosaari (1982).
17. Kajosaari and Saarinen (1983).
18. Businco *et al.* (1983).
19. RCP/BNF Report, p. 19.
20. RCP/BNF Report, p. 25.
21. RCP/BNF Report.
22. RCP/BNF Report, p. 14.
23. RCP/BNF Report, p. 34.
24. Such as some of those described by Warner and Hathaway (1984). Discussed further on p. 66 as I find this very disturbing and dangerous.

Glossary

allergen—substance which causes sensitization, and later, adverse reactions by body tissues.

allergy—the abnormal reaction of sensitized body tissues to the foreign substance of allergen. Clinical immunologists restrict the term to immunological reactions; clinical ecologists use it to describe any adverse reactions.

amino acid—the basic building blocks of protein. 'Essential' ones must be supplied by diet; 'non-essential' ones can be made by the body once it is sufficiently developed.

analgesic—pain-killing.

antibody—protein substance which neutralizes corresponding antigens. Also called immunoglobulin.

antigen—foreign substance able to stimulate the production of antibodies (which is an immune response). All alllergens are antigens, but not vice versa.

areola—darker coloured skin around the nipples.

atopic—having an inherited tendency to develop allergy.

binge—too much of any one substance at any one time. The amount varies as much as the individual.

cell-mediated—an immune response involving particular body cells. There are different types of cells involved, and it's all rather complicated.

coeliac disease—intolerance to gluten, characterized by fat malabsorption and poor growth.

colostrum—fluid produced by mammary glands late in pregnancy or immediately after birth; has very high levels of protective antibodies—a sort of concentrated milk.

'comps'—complementary feeds of artificial formula, water, or 5% glucose; detrimental to lactation and potentially hazardous.

CTL—current tolerance levels—how much the body can presently cope with before symptoms become obvious.

cytotoxic-cell-damaging—Cytotoxic tests measure the damage done to selected blood cells by exposure to known allergens, etc.

double-blind cross-over trial—testing in which the patient is switched between an active treatment and a harmless placebo, with neither the patient nor those attending being aware of which is being given at any time.

endocrine glands—those which secrete hormones.

enuresis—bed-wetting, or involuntary urination.

enzyme—proteins important in body metabolism; they help to bring about various chemical reactions, important in digestion.

excitant—substance which produces a bodily response—in this context, usually adverse—not necessarily mediated by the immune system. Lactose, e.g., would be an excitant for the lactose-intolerant.

fat intolerance—doctors may call this steatorrhea. Characterized by

Food for thought

bulky, pale, offensive loosish stools, which may leave a film of grease floating in the toilet. Common in many cases of food intolerance.

foreign milk—non-specieis-specific; all milks vary greatly from one species to another.

foreign substance—anything that is not part of a particular body, 'non-self'.

gluten—protein found in many cereals, including wheat.

haematuria—blood in urine.

hapten—substance which combines with body protein to form an antigen.

heavy metals—lead, mercury, cadmium, arsenic, etc. Heavy metal pollution is a by-product of industry, and of growing concern.

histamine—chemical released during allergic reactions; also found in some foods, e.g., red wine. Contracts smooth muscle, etc, etc. Anti-histamines block its reaction.

hormone—chemical produced by endocrine glands which causes changes in other parts of the body.

hypoglycaemia—low blood sugar.

hypoallergenic—low allergy, hypo = low; hyper = high.

immune complex—insoluble complex formed when antigen and antibody lock together; may travel via blood or lymph and be deposited in any part of the body, particularly joints.

immune deficiency—deficiency in any part of the immune system whether in the production or interaction of cells or other factors which regulate the immune reaction.

immunity—state of resistance to infection due to the existence of primed antibodies, present since the body's earlier exposure to the antigen.

immunoglobulin—antibody. There are various types present in both blood and milk.

inflammation—changes in blood vessels due to tissue damage.

ingestion—taking in of food, etc. In common parlance, swallowing.

inhalant—something breathed in.

intolerance—adverse bodily reaction to some foreign substance, non-immunological response.

—itis—inflammation, NOT necessarily infection.

in utero—in the uterus.

in vitro—in glass, i.e. a test-tube experiment.

in vivo—in life, i.e. an experiment on living creatures.

involution—the process whereby the uterus (or breast) returns to its pre-pregnant (prelactational) state.

lactase—enzyme which splits lactose (—ase always indicates enzyme).

lactose—sugar of milk.

LIF test—leukocyte (white blood cell) inhibition factor test.

malabsorption—defective absorption, which may range from very slight to very severe. Severe malabsorption is obvious; minor malabsorption may take a long time to be detected and effects are subtle.

mastitis—inflammation in the breast. May be infective or obstructive, or both.

mucosa—membranes which secrete mucus. Common site of reactions.

244

Glossary

neonate—newborn.

neurosis—disordered mental function characterized by abnormal emotion, but without loss of appreciation of external reality (which is psychosis).

nutrients—all those things we need to stay alive and grow: protein, fat, etc.

osmolality—osmosis is the process by which a strong solution draws a weaker solution through a membrane (raisins swell as they soak up water). Osmolality is the measure of the strength of a solution. Osmotic diarrhoea occurs when over strong solutions draw water from the cells of the gut itself.

osmosis—process by which a strong solution draws a weak solution to it through a skin or membrane—as when sultanas are soaked, or children drink heavily sugared fluids in diarrhoea.

oxytocin—hormone produced by pituitary gland which contracts muscle in uterus and in breast; needed for involution of the uterus and also for let-down of milk to infant.

pathogenic—disease-causing.

pharynx—back of the throat.

phenylalanine—an essential amino acid; lack of the enzyme needed to handle it leads to phenylketonuria (PKU).

platelet—blood cells concerned with clotting.

prolactin—hormone important in lactation; levels respond to frequency of sucking stimulus.

prostaglandin—chemicals found in body whose role is being researched; they contract smooth muscle and may be implicated in abnormal gut action for instance.

purpura—haemorrhage under the skin—tiny purple spots.

RAST—radio allergo sorbent test—laboratory test on blood, using radioactive molecules to identify particular Ig levels. Extremely controversial.

rhinitis—nose inflammation.

sensitization—process whereby body tissues develop abnormal sensitivity to excitants; involves creating specific antibodies.

sublingual—under the tongue.

TBL—total body load—i.e. the sum of all present excitants.

toxins—poisons.

trace elements—naturally occurring chemical elements whose role in health and diet varies from crucial to unknown. Include zinc, copper, cobalt, selenium.

trauma—injury.

vascular—of the blood vessels (arteries, veins, capillaries).

vulvo vaginitis—inflammation of vulva and vagina.

zoster—shingles.

Index

Index

Index

Index

Index